PROSPECTIVE RATE SETTING

reprinted from

Topics in Health Care Financing

edited by

William L. Dowling, Ph. D.

Aspen Systems Corporation
Germantown, Maryland
1977

Library of Congress Catalog Card Number: 77-18700
ISBN: 0-89443-028
ISSN: 0095-3814

Printed in the United States of America
1 2 3 4 5

Contents

Prospective Rate Setting

Quick-Reference Subject Locator

Foreword

Prospective rate determination in the health care industry appears to be a virtual certainty. The American Hospital Association, the Blue Cross Association and the Federal government have all expressed their approval of this reimbursement concept. Critics of prospective rate determination are few and far between, and when they surface, they are regarded as intellectual midgets or worse. In short, the industry no longer discusses the desirability of prospective rate determination as an alternative to current retrospective cost determination, rather they focus on the effectiveness of alternative forms of prospective rate setting.

To a large degree, adoption of prospective rate determination reflects prior dissatisfaction with retrospective cost reimbursement by both providers and payers. Providers had become increasingly dissatisfied with retrospective cost reimbursement as the proportion of revenue generated from payers with this mode of reimbursement expanded. It soon became obvious that retrospective cost reimbursement did not provide an adequate allowance for capital costs. Limiting reimbursement to historical cost depreciation charges does not provide funding for plant replacement and modernization in an inflation riddled economy such as ours. This problem is compounded by the rapid rate of technological obsolescence that has been characteristic of the health care industry for the past few decades. The result has been an increasing reliance upon debt financing to meet capital funding requirements. This development places a new element of risk into health care delivery operations which has yet to be fully evaluated.

Payers also became disenchanted with retrospective cost reimbursement as the health care cost spiral accelerated with no visible end in sight. Retrospective cost reimbursement, with all of its associated incentives for inefficiency, was singled out as a possible culprit. Translation of this feeling into legislation occurred at the Federal level in the Social Security Amendments of 1972, which provided for the funding of experiments in prospective reimbursement. In addition, nine states have established rate setting organizations which develop prospective rates. It is generally believed this number will double or triple within a few years, since a large number of states are considering forming some organization to control health care costs through the regulation of rates.

The future of voluntary rate setting organizations, such as those in Virginia, Nebraska and Montana, appears clouded. These organizations are potentially in violation of certain provisions contained in the Sherman Anti-Trust Act. Rate setting organizations operating under the auspices of a government agency are not subject to these same provisions.

Given this irrestible movement to prospective reimbursement, decision-relevant information is urgently needed by health care providers, payers and policy makers. A common framework for discussing the concept of prospective rate determination and alternative formats must be presented to permit provider-payer-policy maker dialogue. Empirical validation of results in various prospective payment plans is also necessary if informed decisions are to be made. Finally, providers, especially, need to know what the informational requirements of a prospective reimbursement plan are likely to be now, and five years from now.

This issue of *Topics in Health Care Financing* is, I believe, a first in the literature dealing with prospective rate determination. It compiles and condenses in one volume a significant amount of information that should help the provider, payer and policy maker make better decisions. I commend Bill Dowling for his selection of authors and articles. I trust that you, the readership, will feel the same after you have completed your reading of this volume.

—William O. Cleverley
Senior Editor

Issue Editor:

William L. Dowling, Ph.D.
Director and Associate Professor
Graduate Program in Health Services Administration and Planning
School of Public Health and Community Medicine
University of Washington
Department of Health Services
Seattle, Washington

Authors:

Robert F. Allison, Ph.D.
Assistant Professor
Program and Bureau of Hospital Administration
University of Michigan
Ann Arbor, Michigan

Frank D. Baker
Executive Director
Washington State Hospital Commission
Olympia, Washington

Katherine G. Bauer
Principle Associate
Harvard Center for Community Health and Medical Care
Harvard University
Boston, Massachusetts

William L. Dowling, Ph.D.

Clifton R. Gaus, Sc.D.
Director
Division of Health Insurance Studies
Office of Research and Statistics
Social Security Administration
Washington, D.C.

Fred J. Hellinger, Ph.D.
Economist
Division of Health Insurance Studies
Office of Research and Statistics
Social Security Administration
Washington, D.C.

Armand P. Leco
Senior Vice President
Blue Cross of Rhode Island
Providence, Rhode Island

John F. Tiscornia
Partner, Arthur Anderson and Company
Seattle, Washington
Clinical Assistant Professor
Department of Health Services
School of Public Health and Community Medicine
University of Washington

Introduction

William L. Dowling, Ph.D.

Prospective rate setting, whereby an external authority determines in advance what hospitals can charge or what third parties must pay them, is attracting the interest of policy makers and purchasers, both public and private, as a way to contain the dramatic and persistent rise in hospital costs. About 35 prospective rate-setting systems are currently in operation across the nation—22 operated by Blue Cross plans, 9 by state agencies or commissions, and several by state hospital associations. Tables 1 and 2 list the Blue Cross and state administered systems in operation as of January 1976.

PROMISE AND PRACTICE

Despite its appeal and promise—what could make more sense than asking hospitals to operate within fixed budgets or rates just as we must live within fixed incomes?—prospective rate setting is not a fully tested and proven strategy. Managers and administrators of the systems in operation have found it extremely difficult to determine how to set "fair but tight" rates that will encourage efficiency without detriment to quality or financial viability. They have also found it difficult to convince different third parties to pay the prospective rates they set. In short, the concept of prospective rate setting makes sense, but problems abound when it is applied in practice. This is not to say that solutions should not be sought. So much is wrong with the current methods of reimbursement—from the perspective of hospitals as well as patients and third party purchasers—that something must be done. This issue of *Topics* explores what is being done to provide administrators and financial managers with up-to-date information about the nature of prospective rate setting and how it might affect their institutions.

In the first chapter we discuss the goals of prospective rate setting systems and the various ways such systems are designed, organized, and sponsored. It turns out that the nature of the constraints and/or incentives a

TABLE 1

Blue Cross Plans with Rate Setting or Review Programs as of January, 1976*

State or Area Within State	Name of Blue Cross Plan	Number Short Term General and Other Special Hospitals Covered	Percent Plan Area Population Enrolled in Blue Cross
Connecticut	Connecticut Blue Cross	40	51
Indiana	Indiana Blue Cross	115	38
Kentucky	Blue Cross Hospital Plan	107	43
Missouri:			
Kansas City area	Blue Cross of Kansas City	57	34
New York:	(under state regulations & approvals)		
New York City	Blue Cross-Blue Shield of N.Y.C.	185	73
Upstate	7 upstate plans; as consortium	140	59
North Carolina**	Blue Cross and Blue Shield of N.C.	133	34
Ohio:			
Cincinnati area	Blue Cross of Southwest Ohio	35	59
Oklahoma	Blue Cross and Blue Shield of Oklahoma	40	24
Rhode Island	(with State Office of Budget)		
	Blue Cross of Rhode Island	15	80
Wisconsin	Associated Hospital Service	149	34
Colorado	Colorado Hospital Service	8 (pilot)	36
Michigan	Michigan Hospital Service	12 (pilot)	58
Ohio:			
Cleveland area	Blue Cross of Northeast Ohio	2 (pilot)	56
Pennsylvania:			
Pittsburgh area	Blue Cross of Western Pennsylvania	17 (pilot)	56
Wilkes-Barre Area	Blue Cross of Northeastern Penn.	2 (pilot)	57

Sources: Communication with Blue Cross Association, January 30, 1976. *Hospital Statistics*, 1975 edition. (1974 data from the American Hospital Association Annual Survey.) American Hospital Association, Chicago, 1975. Blue Cross Association Enrollment and Utilization Report, third quarter, 1975.

*Blue Cross plans in Delaware and New Mexico also have rate review and negotiating provisions in their contracts but are not included here because implementation, so far, has been minimal.

**Voluntary compliance.

Reprinted from Bauer, Katharine, G., "Hospital Rate Setting—This Way to Salvation?" In: Zubkoff, M. and Raskin, I. (eds.), *Hospital Cost Containment*, Milbank Fund, 1976 (forthcoming).

particular prospective rate setting system imposes on hospitals, and hence the way managers should respond to it to further their institutions, depend on how it is designed. It's like the income tax laws; we all agree that taxes are necessary, although late in the evening of April 14 we have our doubts. But without question, the more we know about the tax laws, the easier it is to figure out exactly what we owe. That is, by knowing the rules we maximize our objective—to pay only what we owe and nothing more. In like manner, managers can best direct the institutions they are responsible for if they understand both the concept of prospective rate setting and how the concept is applied in actual practice.

TABLE 2

Hospital Rate Setting Activities of State Governments as of December 1975

Name of State	Type of State Agency	Number of Hospitals Covered	Type of Payer Rates Currently Regulated	Estimated Share of Hospital Revenue Affected
Arizona*	Dept. of Health Services	75	Charges to self-pay pts. Blue Cross	85
Colorado	Department of Social Services	89	Medicaid	8
Connecticut	Independent Commission	40	Charges to self-pay pts.	30
Maryland	Independent Commission	54	Blue Cross Charges to self-pay pts.	55
Massachusetts**	Independent Commission (full time commissioners)	133	Medicaid; Charges to self-pay pts. & others	45
New Jersey	Dept. of Health with concurrence Dept. of Insurance	104	Blue Cross Medicaid	55
New York	Dept. of Health with concurrence Dept. of Insurance; recommendation from Blue Cross plans	320	Medicaid Blue Cross	55
Rhode Island	State Budget Director with R.I. Blue Cross	15	Blue Cross Medicare Medicaid	90
Washington	Independent Commission	119	Charges to self-pay pts. Workmen's Compensation	50–55

Sources: Telephone interviews with state agencies, December, 1975; January, 1976; *Hospital Statistics*, 1975 edition, American Hospital Association

*Hospital rate review is mandatory under Arizona law, but compliance is voluntary. (To date there has been almost 100% compliance.)

**The Massachusetts Rate Setting Commission has approval power over the terms of Blue Cross contracts; since the current contract incorporates controls on charges consonant with the state's charge control law for self-pay patients, the 45% figure understates the Commission's overall leverage.

Reprinted from Bauer, Katharine, G., "Hospital Rate Setting—This Way to Salvation?" In: Zubkoff M. and Raskin, I. (eds.), *Hospital Cost Containment*, Milbank Fund, 1976 (forthcoming).

4 HOW?

How are rates actually set in prospective rate setting systems? What information is required of hospitals, and how is it used? What factors are considered? Last year's operating costs? Next year's budget? Expected inflation? New programs? Future capital needs? What process is followed in setting rates? Is some mechanical formula used? Are budgets reviewed, and if so in how much detail? Are rates actually negotiated, when it comes right down to it? And what happens if, during the prospective years, a hospital feels it just cannot manage within its rates? Each of the ongoing prospective rate-setting systems deals with these questions in a different way, as there is no prototype system—no one best way. Nevertheless, Armand Leco, Senior Vice President of Rhode Island's Blue Cross Plans, and Frank Baker, Executive Director of the Washington State Hospital Commission, provide a considerable insight by discussing candidly how their systems handle these issues. They describe their prospective rate setting programs in detail with emphasis on the "nitty-gritty"—how they really work.

Rhode Island

In the Rhode Island system, budgets are negotiated on a one-to-one basis between Blue Cross and each hospital, but within a statewide "maxi-cap"—an aggregate cost increase ceiling for all hospitals for the coming year which is negotiated by Blue Cross, the Hospital Association of Rhode Island, and the state, before the individual budget negotiations take place. Each hospital attempts to negotiate what it believes to be its financial needs for the coming year, but in the aggregate, the budgets Blue Cross agrees to must fall within the maxi-cap. This is a very unique system, and one that is attracting a lot of interest. In Rhode Island, for example, Medicare and Medicaid—which in the final analysis are concerned about the aggregate expenditures or expenditure increases from year to year, not the rates they pay for specific services—are willing to waive their principles of reimbursement and pay whatever rates are negotiated for individual hospitals, as long as they feel that the maxi-cap is reasonable, since it guarantees a ceiling to their payments to hospitals for the coming year. Intriguing also is the way the rate setting program in Rhode Island takes into account the priorities the state's planning agency assigns to approved new services.

Washington

In Washington, where rates are set by a public utility type commission and each hospital's budget is judged in comparison to the budgets of its peers, things are quite different. All hospitals are required to use a uniform chart of acounts, uniform accounting, uniform budgeting, and uniform financial reporting—a requirement which many believe is inevitable everywhere. Budgeted costs are "screened" against aggregate indicators of reasonableness—total cost per case and per day, and ancillary, routine, and support costs per case and per day. If a budget fails these screens, it is subjected to more detailed screens—like the cost per unit of output in specific departments. Only if a budget fails these screens is it reviewed in detail, line by line, if necessary. Intriguing about this approach is that administrators know that if they submit a budget that is not out of line with their peers, there will be no line by line review, no "second-guessing" of management decisons and plans, no challenging of management prerogatives. The Washington system attempts to deal explicitly with the full financial requirements of hospitals including future capital needs, but within the context of long-range plans. Both systems are unique in many ways, since as noted above, there is little agreement at this time on how to handle the many issues surrounding rate setting. Yet these two systems are among the most refined, and between them they capture most of the elements of rate setting found in the other systems.

VOICES OF EXPERIENCE

What has been the experience of the prospective rate-setting systems currently in operation? Have they contained cost increases? Have they impacted on the quality or financial viability of the hospitals subject to them? Clifton Gaus and Fred Hellinger, of the Social Security Administration's Office of Research and Statistics, give some answers to these and other equally important questions in their article summarizing the findings of five SSA-sponsored evaluations of ongoing prospective rate-setting systems. It turns out that cost savings appear modest. But what does this mean? Is this approach to reimbursement not all it's alleged to be, or are there design flaws, due perhaps to the newness of the strategy and the difficulty of designing a system in which all of the constraints and/or incentives operate in the right direction? Can prospective rate setting in and of itself correct all of the problems that exist in the delivery of hospital services, or must it be better coordinated with complimentary programs like planning and utilization review? Reading this introduction leads one to the conclusion that we have a lot to learn. Where better to begin, however, for both managers and rate setters than the experience of the prospective rate-setting systems that are actually in operation. It should be noted, too, that not only is SSA assisting many prospective rate-setting systems in one way or another, but it has also indicated its willingness to waive the Medicare reimbursement regulations in order to participate in such systems, where they appear able to set fair but tight rates. A number of state Medicaid programs are saying the same thing.

Administrative Reaction

How do administrators actually react to prospective rate setting? Robert Allison, who is conducting an evaluation of Michigan Blue Cross' system—a system which establishes a total budget within which hospitals must operate for the coming year, rather than setting per diem or per specific service rates, as most prospective rate setting systems do—provides insight into this question. What area of costs do administrators believe they can actually control? In comparison, and perhaps in contrast, what areas appear to offer the largest cost savings potential? How are budgeting and control practices affected? How are department heads involved? And what about administrator-medical staff relations; how are they affected by cost-containment efforts? Allison reports how administrators actually feel about the cost-saving possibilities *and* realities they face when subject to a prospective rate-setting system.

Preparation

John Tiscornia, a Partner in the Seattle office of Arthur Andersen and Company, offers advice about what managers should be doing to prepare their institutions for or to actually function under prospective rate setting. Drawing on many years as an adviser to hospitals in the area of financial management, he describes how prospective rate setting can affect hospitals, not in theory but in practice. What changes in accounting and financial management practices can be expected? How will budgeting and pricing be affected? Will prospective rate setting reduce management flexibility and discretion? What operational problems can be expected, and how can they best be dealt with? More important, how do administrators and financial managers prepare their governing boards and management teams for prospective rate setting? And most important perhaps, how might prospective rate setting impact on the long run financial viability of their institutions?

Data for Decisions

Katharine Bauer, who has examined the promise and the practice of rate setting more thoroughly than anyone else, discusses the information required for rate setting (and for planning, because as it turns out, the two are inevitably interrelated). Based on a study she made of the data collected and reported by rate setting agencies and programs, few rate setting officials feel that the data available to them are sufficient for the judgments they should be making. More data then are likely to be sought from hospitals. However, the first step is to determine the uses to which such data would be put so that demands are not unjustified. And, it appears that most of the data needed could be obtained from existing sources, if efforts are made to do so. More data! Now that can be viewed by administrators and financial managers in two ways. As an additional burden. Or, as an opportunity to get data they probably should be using anyway for management planning and control purposes. Either way, it is important that managers begin to gear their data systems to answer the questions about the efficiency and efficacy of their institutions that rate setting officials will surely be asking in the not too distant future.

1

Prospective Rate Setting: Concept and Practice

William L. Dowling, Ph.D.

Topics in this chapter include:

WHAT IS PROSPECTIVE RATE SETTING?

PROSPECTIVE RATE SETTING is a cost containment strategy wherein an external authority establishes the prices that providers are allowed to charge and/or that third parties are required to pay for specified services in advance of the period in which the services are actually provided. To the extent that patients and third parties do in fact pay the prospectively set rates, prospective rate setting might more appropriately be called prospective rate payment, or just prospective payment. The key difference between prospective payment (or prospective reimbursement as it is often called) and conventional forms of reimbursement is that providers are not paid the costs they actually incur in providing the services being paid for, nor are they free to unilaterally adjust their charges to cover these costs; rather, providers are paid at rates set in advance of and considered fixed for the pertinent period (typically a year). Although costs are not constrained directly under prospective payment, it is assumed that the constraint on revenue imposed by fixing provider charges and/or third party payment rates in advance of the prospective year will cause providers to contain their costs during that year in order to avoid losses (or earn surpluses).

Prospective rate setting differs from retrospective cost reimbursement in that payment rates are specified in advance rather than determined after the fact and are not based on costs actually incurred during the prospective year. Prospective rate setting differs from institutional rate setting in that an external authority is involved and has the final say regarding rates. Providers are not free to set their rates initially or to change them during the prospective year, without going through some sort of review and approval process. Prospective payment systems are designed to introduce marketplace-like financial incentives into the provider sector. Providers face firm fixed prices for their services. If they are able to keep their costs below these prices, they will make a surplus; if not, they will suffer a loss. Thus, providers are definitely at risk.

The basic elements of prospective rate setting, then, are simple:

1. An external authority is empowered (by statute, market power, or voluntary compliance by providers) to set provider charges and/or third party payment rates.
2. Rates are set in advance of the prospective year during which they apply and are considered fixed for the year (except for major, uncontrollable, unpredictable occurrences).
3. Patients and/or third parties pay the prospective rates rather than the costs actually incurred by providers during the year (or charges adjusted to cover these costs).
4. Providers are at risk for losses or surpluses.

A particular prospective rate setting system may only approximate these elements in actual practice. For example, a rate setting agency or program may see itself as "reviewing and approving" rather than "setting" provider rates; that is, the stringency of the rate determination process and the range of factors considered can vary greatly. The prospectively set rates may be paid only by self-pay patients, or by Blue Cross, or Medicaid, or all three; that is, the applicability of the rates can vary. The prospectively set rates may be adjusted automatically for specified factors like the actual case mix, inflation, volume, etc., experienced by providers during the prospective year, or adjustments may be made so readily upon provider request at the end of the prospective year that most of the risk associated with advance rate setting is eliminated. Or, what amounts to the same thing, any losses or surpluses providers make may be compensated for or taken away in the following year's rates. Hence, the term "prospective" must be applied with care to any particular rate setting system, depending on how closely it approaches the "spirit" as well as the "letter" of the concept of prospectivity.

WHY PROSPECTIVE RATE SETTING?

Prospective rate setting evolved in response to the dramatic and persistent rise in hospital costs that began in the mid-1960s. It was then (and continues to be) widely believed that the cost inflation problem can be traced to an absence of cost containment incentives in the prevailing methods of paying hospitals—the payment of costs (determined retrospectively) and the payment of billed changes (set unilaterally by institutions themselves). Prospective rate setting was seen both as a means of exerting more external influence over hospital activities and plans, and as a means of building cost containment constraints and/or incentives into hospital payment. All prospective rate setting systems claim cost containment as a primary objective. State rate setting laws, for example, typically assign an agency or commission the job of assuring that hospital rates reflect "the costs of efficient production of services" or "the economy-wide inflation rate," or that they are, simply, "reasonable." The range of cost-influencing factors considered in judging the reasonableness of rates varies greatly, however. Some rate-setting systems focus on per unit costs, emphasizing efficiency or productivity; others look more broadly at aggregate hospital costs, emphasizing efficiency and utilization; others look even more broadly at aggregate system costs, emphasizing efficiency, utilization, and the supply of beds, facilities, and services. In general, rate setting agencies and programs also recognize the need to preserve the ability of hospitals to provide quality care and to remain financially viable.

In general, rate setting agencies and programs recognize the need to preserve the ability of hospitals to provide quality care and to remain financially viable.

In a number of states, hospitals acted through their associations to encourage the development of prospective rate setting systems, hoping that impartial rate setting authorities would come to agree with them that the cost inflation problem was largely attributable to factors beyond their control. These authorities might help explain this to the public and might even serve as advocates for hospitals with regard to certain of their financial problems. In addition, hospitals hoped that all third parties would be willing to pay rates set by independent rate setting agencies or programs, thereby ending the imposition by the different third parties of arbitrary cost or rate ceilings, different definitions of allowable costs, and different reimbursement practices. This, in turn, would help hospitals achieve the goal of "equal payment for equal services" and end the practice of shifting costs not reimbursed by third parties to self-pay patients. Both hospitals and third parties believed they would benefit from the financial predictability prospective rate setting makes possible.

MANAGEMENT IMPLICATIONS

Proponents of prospective rate setting believe that the financial incentives inherent in this approach to payment (i.e., the possibility of a loss or surplus) will cause providers[1] to give costs more weight in decision making with regard to current operations and future plans. Prospective rate setting makes it essential for hospitals to accurately budget and effectively justify their anticipated expenditures for the coming year, since prospective rates are generally based in some way on a budget review. Even in rate setting systems where budgets are not used in rate setting (e.g., those in which a formula is used to project historical costs into prospective rates), budgets are fundamental to rate appeals and end-of-year reviews. In addition to providing a way to demonstrate a hospital's financial requirements, accurate budgeting becomes critical for self protection. If costs increase more than anticipated in a hospital's budget, its prospective rates may not generate sufficient revenue to cover its costs. Hence, prospective rate setting should lead to better budgeting practices.

Demonstrate Need

Prospective rate setting also makes it essential for hospitals to demonstrate the need for any new facilities and services to be added during the prospective year and to accurately forecast the additional costs associated with them, since this is the first step in attempting to assure that prospective rates cover the costs of new services. Detailed capital and program cost studies are commonly required to demonstrate the need for requested rates. However, even in rate setting systems where rates are not based directly on the costing-out of specific programs and services (e.g., in formula schemes), accurate cost studies are important as a basis for appeals, or (where a hospital fails to obtain approval for what it requests) as a basis for internal decisions regarding planning priorities and trade-offs. For example, management might be forced to ask: "If we can count on only so much revenue given our prospective rates, is it more important to provide service x or service y given the costs and benefits of each?" Under stringent prospective payment systems, program budgeting may advance rapidly to a state where alternative program possibilities can be examined by means of budget models to estimate their cost and revenue implications before implementation decisions are made. Capital and program plans may also come to be used in prospective rate-setting systems as a basis for decisions regarding how much "growth and development" to allow hospitals to enable them to accumulate the capital reserves that would be needed in future years to implement their long-range plans. For these reasons, prospective rate setting should lead to better capital and program planning.

Cost Controls

Prospective rate setting also makes it essential to understand the cost implications of the quantity, quality, intensity, and scope of services offered, and to closely monitor these aspects of operation. Under stringent prospective payment systems, prompt adjustments in these and other cost-influencing factors may have to be made during the prospective year in attempting to control costs to keep them within prospective rates. Hence, prospective rate setting should lead to better cost analysis and cost control techniques. It appears that the amount of influence administrators and financial managers exert in organizational decision-making will continue to grow as a greater premium is placed on their planning and control skills. In addition, the scope of their influence should broaden as tightening financial constraints make it essential to recognize and act on the cost and revenue implications of everything from productivity and purchasing to the case mix of patients treated and the services they receive.

Sophistication

In short, management sophistication will improve substantially under prospective rate setting as it becomes more difficult for high-cost hospitals to bail themselves out by raising rates or by expecting cost reimbursement to cover whatever they spend. In addition, since the laws creating state rate setting systems and the policies guiding voluntary programs typically call for the setting of rates related to "the costs of efficient production" and typically recognize the need to maintain "financial viability," it can be anticipated that new demands will be placed on accounting and financial reporting systems to produce the information required to demonstrate "efficiency" and "financial viability." This information will be used more and more in rate setting and in appeals. Parenthetically, financial ratio analysis should emerge as a more important management tool.

ANALYTICS OF PROSPECTIVE RATE SETTING

Cost-Volume-Revenue

The financial incentives and implications of prospective rate setting can be analyzed by means of a conventional break-even model. Figure 1a is a graphic presentation of the cost-revenue-volume relationships for a hypothetical hospital. Output volume is measured along the horizontal axis (in discharges, days, or services) and costs and revenues along the vertical axis. Suppose the hospital's

FIGURE 1A. COST-REVENUE-VOLUME RELATIONSHIP

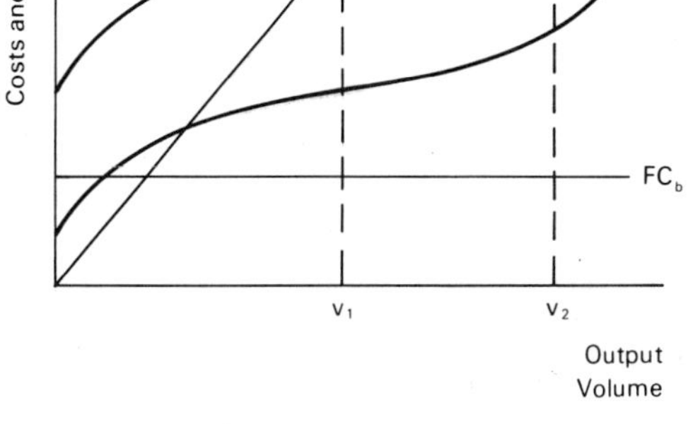

FIGURE 1B. SIMPLIFIED COST-REVENUE-VOLUME RELATIONSHIP

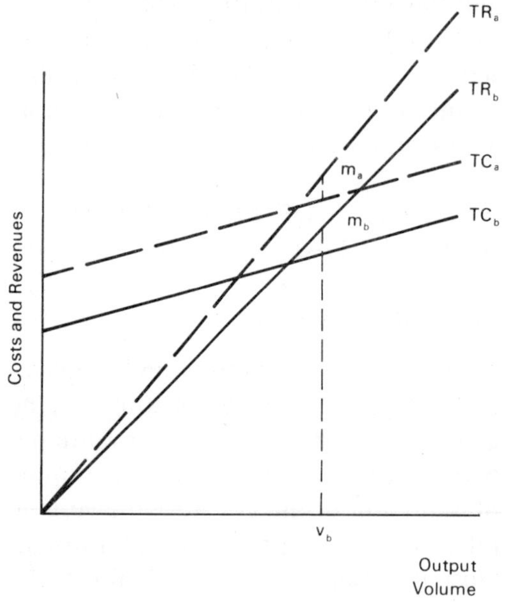

budgeted fixed and variable costs at different possible volumes are shown by the curves FC_b and VC_b, giving budgeted total costs at different possible volumes of TC_b. Assuming that both self-pay patients and third parties pay fixed charges or rates per unit of service, budgeted total revenue would increase in direct proportion to volume as shown by the straight line TR_b. In actual practice, of course, costs and revenues are only budgeted for some relevant range of volume like $v_1 - v_2$.

Figure 1b is a simplified version of Figure 1a, showing the hospital's TC_b and TR_b approximated by straight lines. In the absence of prospective rate setting or any other constraint on charges, the hospital would presumably set its charges so that TR_b would exceed TC_b by some desired operating margin, m_b, at its expected volume, v_b. If actual volume equals expected volume and the hospital's expectations about costs and revenues are right, the hospital would end the year with an actual operating margin of m_b. If actual costs begin running higher than expected as shown by TC_a, the hospital would presumably increase its charges during the year (again assuming no constraint on rate setting) to a level that would generate total revenue TR_a and operating margin m_a ($m_a = m_b$). This illustrates why it is felt that billed charges payment systems, in which hospitals are free to increase their charges at will, fail to provide cost containment incentives. Rather than finding ways to prevent costs from increasing more than expected, hospitals can just increase their charges to cover them. From Figure 1b, it can also be seen that if actual volume turns out to be greater than expected volume, the hospital would end up with an operating margin greater than m_a or m_b whether TC_a and TR_a or TC_b and TR_b apply. This illustrates why it is felt that billed charges payment systems encourage increases in utilization. The greater the volume, the greater the operating margin.

Retrospective Reimbursement

Figure 2 illustrates the financial situation of a hypothetical hospital under retrospective cost reimbursement. Abstracting from the realities of nonallowable costs and nonrecognized financial requirements, and assuming for simplicity that all revenue comes in the form

FIGURE 2. RETROSPECTIVE COST REIMBURSEMENT

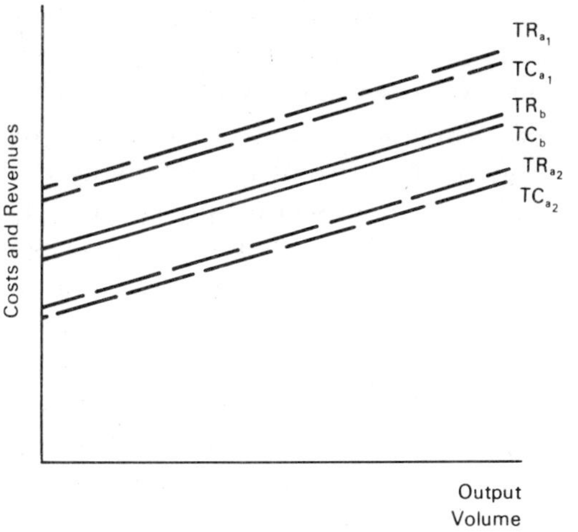

of cost reimbursement, this method of payment means that the hospital's revenues would always just equal its costs, whatever they happen to be (i.e., TR and TC would be the same). If actual costs begin running higher than expected as shown by TC_{a_1}, the hospital's revenue would still cover its costs as shown by TR_{a_1}, since payment is based on costs. On the other hand, if the hospital contained its costs to TC_{a_2}, it would only receive revenue TR_{a_2}. This illustrates why cost reimbursement is so often criticized as a scheme under which "whatever a hospital spends, it gets back." Clearly, cost reimbursement fails to provide cost containment incentives; hospitals are neither penalized for cost increases or rewarded for finding ways to prevent them.

Incentives Contrast

The financial incentives inherent in prospective rate setting contrast sharply with those of the conventional methods of reimbursement. Suppose a prospective rate setting system sets per case, per day, or per specific services rates for each participating hospital at a level just high enough to generate sufficient revenue to cover the hospital's approved budgeted costs and provide an agreed upon operating margin at the expected output volume. Figure 3 illustrates this situation for a hypothetical hospital. TC_b represents the hospital's approved budgeted costs, TR_{pr} the revenue that the hospital's prospective rates will generate at different output volumes, m_b the agreed upon operating margin, and v_b the expected volume. Note that the hospital's rates are set in advance of the prospective year based on budgeted vs. actual costs, with the hospital's budget first reviewed for reasonableness. Once set, the hospital's rates are considered fixed for the year.

FIGURE 3. PROSPECTIVE PAYMENT

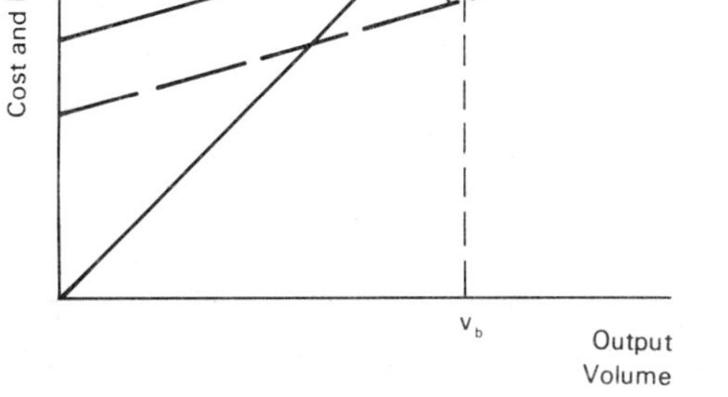

Suppose the hospital's actual costs for the year exceed its approved budgeted costs as shown by TC_{a_1}. Under a prospective payment system, the hospital would suffer a loss equal to l, since it would not be free to increase its rates. On the other hand, if the hospital is able to contain its costs to TC_{a_2}, it would earn a surplus s, substantially greater than the agreed-to operating margin m_b. In contrast to both billed charges systems (where hospitals are free to set their own charges) and cost reimbursement systems, prospective payment systems provide a penalty for greater than expected cost increases. Higher costs mean financial losses. Thus, once a hospital's prospective rate is set, it faces a strong "negative incentive" to keep its costs below its rate. In contrast to cost reimbursement systems (where containing costs results in less revenue) prospective payment systems provide a "positive incentive" to keep costs down—the possibility of earning a surplus.

It should be noted, however, that it is not clear why a nonprofit hospital would prefer to contain its costs during the prospective year in order to earn a surplus to spend in future years. Why wouldn't it simply spend whatever it wishes each and every year (which a hospital theoretically could do under charges or cost reimbursement)? What is the advantage, in other words, of deferred spending? This is one of the key issues surrounding prospective rate setting. Some observers argue that prospective rate setting really offers no positive incentive to hospitals (at least, not to nonprofit hospitals which cannot distribute surpluses to their owners), since by cutting costs to earn a surplus, a hospital is just putting off expenditures it could make during the prospective year while risking lower rates in future years. It does appear that the negative incentive of the possibility of a loss must be present for prospective rate setting to work. However, some observers argue that the positive incentive inherent in prospective rate setting should be emphasized more. Prospective rates should be set so that efficient hospitals can make a surplus. Surpluses so acquired should place hospitals able to make them in an advantageous position with regard to some objectives they value. For example, planning agencies might place more emphasis on the cost of capital in considering competing expansion, modernization, or new service proposals. If several hospitals are seeking approval to add a particular new service, perhaps approval should be given to the one that could finance the project most cheaply as a result of its ability to accumulate enough surplus to obviate the need to borrow and incur debt service expenses.

Efficiency

Whether the planning process is formally structured along these lines, some proponents of prospective rate setting argue that over time efficient hospitals would find it easier than inefficient hospitals to keep their costs below their rates, and would, therefore, be more likely to expand (perhaps using accumulated surpluses). Inefficient hospitals would tend to suffer losses, forcing them to curtail their operations. Thus, there would be a gradual shift from less efficient to more efficient hospitals in the long run. This argument assumes that prospective payment systems can be designed to be sufficiently sensitive to reward efficient hospitals (which may not necessarily have the lowest costs) and penalize inefficient hospitals (which may not have the highest costs). It is not clear, however, that the prospective payment systems currently in operation are sophisticated enough to discriminate between efficient and inefficient hospitals. In large part, the problem is caused by an inability to measure output mix and quality accurately enough to know when a hospital's costs are unjustifiably out of line.

Present Status

At the present time, about 35 prospective rate setting systems are in operation. Twenty-two Blue Cross plans operate prospective rate review or rate setting programs. Most of these involve all hospitals in the plan's region or state, but a few are small experiments involving only a few hospitals. Nine states have enacted rate setting laws. In four, an independent public utility form of rate setting commission has been set up; in the other five, rate setting is performed by an existing agency of government, typically the department of health. In three states, state hospital associations operate voluntary rate review programs, and the University of South Carolina operates an experimental program with 16 hospitals.

These prospective rate setting systems are far from uniform. They differ not only with regard to the sponsoring organization, as indicated above, but also with regard to the nature of the prospective rates, the method of rate setting used, the extent to which different third parties actually pay the rates, and other factors.

SPONSORSHIP

The agency or organization sponsoring prospective rate setting may well affect the stringency of the system. Participation by hospitals in Blue Cross and state hospital association programs is generally voluntary, whereas participation in state systems is mandatory; and it is reasonable to expect that programs lacking the authority to require participation are not likely to be as stringent as mandatory systems. Governing boards, given their trusteeship responsibility, cannot be expected to voluntarily subject their hospitals to financial risk. Their duty to protect the financial viability of the institutions simply runs counter to their concept of employing financial risk to encourage cost containment. Only hospitals that believe prospective payment will not detract from the achievement of their goals or the maintenance of their financial viability can be expected to join, if given a choice, and any hospital adversely affected can be expected to drop out, if this is possible. Therefore, the impact of voluntary rate setting systems would likely be less substantial than mandatory systems. This line of reasoning has led many to prefer state sponsored systems.

It should be recognized, however, that prospective rate setting was first pioneered by several Blue Cross plans, and

The impact of voluntary rate setting systems would likely be less substantial than mandatory systems. This line of reasoning has led many to prefer state sponsored systems.

in specific situations, an arm's length but positive relationship with hospitals, expertise, market power, personalities, and a shared concern for cost containment have combined to produce effective Blue Cross programs. In comparison to state agencies, Blue Cross programs tend to be better staffed, more flexible, freer to experiment, freer to negotiate, and less encumbered by regulatory red tape. In the final analysis, however, Blue Cross rate setting programs are voluntary, and any program seen as too stringent might end up without any takers. In addition, hospitals can always threaten to cancel their Blue Cross contracts, although some plans cover such a large share of the market that such an action is hardly likely. Hospital association sponsored prospective rate review programs inevitably suffer a credibility problem, although several associations, guided by strong leadership and motivated by the threat of state regulation have developed extensive budget and rate review programs.

MANDATORY PROGRAMS

Mandatory rate setting programs are created by the enactment of state laws empowering an existing state agency such as the state department of health or one created especially for the purpose, such as an independent public utility type rate setting commission to set rates for hospitals (and in some cases, for nursing facilities and other institutional providers as well). State laws generally require hospitals to provide any data requested by the agency or commission in the format specified. State laws may or may not require the different third parties to pay the approved rates. Hence, there are states in which the rates apply only to patients who pay billed charges with Blue Cross and Medicaid continuing to reimburse costs. In other states, Blue Cross and Medicaid are required to pay the approved rates. No state, of course, has jurisdiction over the Federal Medicare program, but in Maryland, Rhode Island, Washington, and Western Pennsylvania, the Social Security Administration has waived certain of the Medicare reimbursement principles in order to participate in operating prospective payment systems. The question of who pays the prospectively set rates in a particular system is important, of course, because the greater the proportion of a hospital's revenue coming in the form of prospective rate payment, the greater the impact the system is likely to have. In addition, the "equal payment for equal services" goal requires that all patients and third parties pay the prospective rates set by the agency or program, although the issue of how to handle cost differences experienced by hospitals because of differences in third party policies and practices (and hence whether different rates should be permitted) is far from settled.

Of the two state alternatives, the department of health or an independent rate setting commission, hospitals generally prefer the latter, arguing that a conflict of interest exists when the agency administering the state's Medicaid program and hence purchasing large amounts of hospital services is also empowered to set the rates to be paid for these services. Commissions are also considered freer from political influence than agencies of state government, although in actual practice their budgets are usually determined annually by the legislature. State agencies and independent commissions alike often suffer from underfinancing, understaffing, and inflexible procedures.

ADVANTAGES

Could the advantages of both private and state sponsorship be gained in a rate setting program cooperatively sponsored by a Blue Cross plan or hospital association and a state agency or commission? This possibility merits further investigation. The authority to set rates and to mandate participation could come from a state law while administration of the program, including the actual budget review and rate setting process, could be carried out by the private organization. The state might finally approve all rates, acting upon the recommendation of the review organization, or it might establish a state-wide ceiling on aggregate costs within which the private organization would be free to work out specific rates for individual hospitals. In New York and Rhode Island, Blue Cross plans operate prospective rate setting programs within the framework of regulations promulgated by the respective states. The plans administer the rate setting process and recommend rates and rate appeal settlements to the appropriate state agency.

PLANNING AND RATE SETTING

Another fundamental issue is whether certification of need, licensure, and other regulatory functions should be placed in the agency that handles rate setting or be kept separate. No state has given all of these powers to an independent rate setting commission, and although in a number of states where rate setting has been assigned to the department of health, the department carries out the certificate of need and licensure functions as well, there is surprisingly little coordination between them. Reflecting the lack of coherent state (or national) health policies, no state has a truly comprehensive, cohesive regulatory program at this time. In part, this may stem from an unwillingness of states to face up to the effect of their own decisions granting certificates of need, or raising licensure standards, or expanding Medicaid eligibility and services on costs and hence on rates. Examples can be found of states in which the state's Medicaid program is unwilling to pay the prospective rates set by the state's own rate setting commission as fair and reasonable. It should be noted, however, that some prefer the problems caused by multiple, uncoordinated, often conflicting regulatory and payment programs to the centralization of programs and hence power in a single agency.

Spiraling Cost

Perhaps the most fundamental question is whether the cost spiral can ever be dealt with definitively until financing, planning, licensing, utilization and rate setting programs are linked. Clearly, for example, the scope and sophistication of facilities and services offered by hospitals affect costs, and it is generally agreed that decisions about the appropriateness of existing or new services should be based on both cost and need criteria. It seems only fair, however, that once approvals for new services are given, they carry with them authority to adjust rates to cover the costs of these services. Likewise, costs should be considered in determining the eligibility limits and the services to be provided in programs that finance care for the needy, but once services are promised, they should be paid for. In the final analysis, it is the inevitability of making cost availability-accessability-quality tradeoff decisions such as these that argues both for coordinating the different financing and regulatory programs that deal with these matters and for placing them in public agencies where such decisions can be legitimized in the public interest.

Certainly, the rate setting agency should expect help from planning agencies in encouraging the sharing of services to improve operating efficiency.

Coordination

Coordination of planning and rate setting remains an illusive goal, although some steps have been taken. It has become commonplace, for example, to require planning agency approval before the capital costs, and in some cases the operating costs, of new services are figured into payment rates. Another coordination mechanism operating in several states is where the rate setting agency or commission advises planning agencies regarding the reasonableness of the capital and operating costs as well as the financial feasibility of proposed projects. It has been suggested that the rate setting agency might even suggest a state-wide ceiling on capital expenditures each year, with only the highest priority new services (as determined by planning agencies) implemented up to the point at which the ceiling is reached. Certainly, the rate setting agency should expect help from planning agencies in encouraging the sharing of services to improve operating efficiency.

It has also been suggested that the powers of rate setting be brought to bear to back up the decisions of planning agencies. For example, if an area is found to be overbedded by the appropriate planning agency, the prospective routine daily service rates for area hospitals could be based on what per diem costs would be at efficient occupancy levels rather than on what they are at actual occupancy levels, thereby forcing the closure of beds or merger of units to avoid financial losses. In Massachusetts and New York, for example, prospective rates are adjusted to penalize hospitals with obstetrics units operating under 60 percent occupancy, pediatrics units under 70 percent, and medical-surgical units under 80 percent. This approach could be taken to force the phase-out of any specialized service declared to be duplicative and underutilized on the grounds that rates are to be set so as to cover the costs of "efficient" provision, not low volume provision, of services. Certainly, rate setting should be flexible enough to support the efforts of planning agencies to promote alternatives to acute inpatient care, cooperation in the provision of services, regionalization, etc. An intriguing possibility, just beginning to receive attention, is the concept of relating the amount allowed in hospital rates for depreciation (or growth and development) to future area needs and approved institutional long range plans. It has been suggested, for example, that hospitals in overbedded areas should not automatically be guaranteed the financial means to replace themselves, while hospitals that are clearly needed should be allowed more than historical depreciation to enable them to accumulate the capital revenues they will need in future years.

BASIS OF PAYMENT

Prospective rate setting systems differ in terms of the basis or unit of payment for which rates are set. This feature is important because the payment unit determines the incentiv tem and hence how hospitals are likely to react to it. The alternative bases of payment that might be used are as follows:

1. Apportionment of total budget
2. Apportionment of departmental budgets
3. Capitation
4. Case
5. Day
6. Specific services

Total Budget

The apportionment of total budget method might work in the following way. Hospitals would submit budgets to a rate setting agency or program setting forth and justifying their expected prospective year costs and financial requirements. The agency would assess the reasonableness of each hospital's budget, perhaps by comparing its costs to the costs of similar hospitals, to cost standards, to expected inflation trends, or by a line by line budget review. Hospitals would be asked to defend or modify any parts of their budgets appearing out of line. Agreement on a final budget satisfactory to both parties might be automatic if a budget, as originally submitted or as modified, fell within acceptable parameters, or agreement might be reached through a formal hearings process, an informal negotiations process, or a combination of the two. Once a hospital's budget was agreed upon, each third party would be obligated to pay its share of budgeted costs, regardless (following the basic principle of prospective payment) of the costs actually incurred by the hospital during the prospective year. Apportionment of budgeted costs to different third parties could be based on each third party's share of the hospital's charges, admissions, or patient days, or could be determined by the departmental RCC method (applied to budgeted vs. actual costs). The hospital would be guaranteed its budgeted costs whatever the proportions paid by the different third parties. For example, if a budget of $6,000,000 were agreed upon for a hospital, the hospital would get this amount regardless of what its costs actually turned out to be. If a particular third party were responsible for half the hospital's patients, it would be obligated to pay $3,000,000 (which it might simply forward in monthly $250,000 installments). Quarterly checks could be made to determine each third party's exact share of the $2,000,000 due the hospital for the quarter.

Michigan Blue Cross and Washington's State Hospital Commission are currently experimenting with the apportionment of budget method of prospective payment. Military and Veteran's Administration hospitals and hospitals in a number of Canadian provinces essentially operate on fixed budgets set in advance of each operating year. Obviously, this approach to prospective payment provides an incentive to control both the cost per unit and volume of services provided, since both contribute to the total cost of operating an institution. In actual practice, provision would undoubtedly be made to adjust the budgeted cost figure agreed to for a hospital, if its actual costs or volume diverge substantially from its budgeted costs because of major, uncontrollable, unpredictable occurrences. It merits repeating, however, that automatically adjusting what a hospital is paid based on how it actually operates during the prospective year removes the incentive to control operations.

Departmental Budgets

The apportionment of departmental budgets method of prospective payment is similar, except that cost figures are set for individual departments, and each third party's payment responsibility is determined by the proportion of each department's services going to its patients. The advantage of this approach is the "fine tuning" it makes possible in focusing financial incentives on specific areas of operation. In addition, it allows the elimination of departments over which the administrator has little or no control from prospective rate setting. Or, only the routine daily service and "hotel" cost centers might be included under the assumption that their costs are less influenced by changes in case mix, intensity of service, technology, etc., than the ancillary cost centers. The Connecticut Hospital Association has experimented with a modified version of the departmental budgets method in setting cost targets.

Capitation

The capitation method of prospective payment, as an approach to hospital vs. physician payment, would work best where hospitals are associated with or part of health plans or health maintenance organizations. Each hospital would agree to provide to the enrollees of the plan with which it is associated all needed hospital services in return for a fixed amount per person per year. Although it is conceivable that the capitation approach to payment could be used for hospitals not associated with health plans, this would require that groups of people in areas served by one or more hospitals identify themselves with specific hospitals that would accept responsibility for meeting their hospital needs. It is difficult to see how this would work in metropolitan areas. People do not identify directly with hospitals as they do with physicians, and so it would be difficult to determine which hospital was responsible for which people unless physicians were involved. Nevertheless, in a 1964 experiment conducted by Colorado Blue Cross in Yuma County, Colorado, the Plan made capitation payments to the two hospitals in the County which in turn agreed to provide all hospital services needed by Blue Cross subscribers. Yuma County is quite isolated, however, and each hospital's share of Blue Cross' business in the County was well known.

Per Case, Per Diem

Per case, per diem, or per specific services prospective rates are more familiar. The actual determination of per unit rates can be done by dividing approved budgeted costs by expected volume, or by asking hospitals to propose rate structures that will generate just enough revenue to cover approved budgeted costs at expected volumes, or by applying some sort of formula to project historical costs forward into prospective rates or to translate hospital and patient workload characteristics into prospective rates. The only operating per case rate prospective payment program is an experiment being conducted by Blue Cross of Northeastern Pennsylvania with two hospitals in Wilkes-Barre. However, Phase IV of the Economic Stabilization Program, which of course was never implemented because of the termination of the Program, would have employed as its basic cost control mechanism a limit of 7.5 percent on annual increases in revenue per case. In the prospective rate setting programs sponsored by Blue Cross plans, choice of a payment unit generally follows the approach to reimbursement that the plan used before. Thus, plans that reimbursed costs tend to set per diem prospective rates, and plans that paid billed charges tend to set specific services rates.

Specific Services

A practical advantage of using specific services as the bases of payment is that services represent a common denominator applicable to all purchasers of hospital services—Blue Cross, commercial insurance, self-pay patients, Medicare, Medicaid, etc. Third parties reimbursing hospitals all-inclusive per diem costs tend to prefer per diem prospective rates. However, it would be inappropriate to charge individual self-pay patients average per diem rates, since some would end up paying for much more service than they actually used and some for less. Therefore, either a dual rate structure would be required to satisfy third parties and individual self-pay patients, or all purchasers would have to agree on specific services as the basis of payment. State commissions, concerned about getting all purchasers to pay the same rates for the same services, seem to favor specific services rates, and several commissions have attempted to get Medicare and Medicaid to waive their cost reimbursement regulations and agree to pay the rates they set. Another advantage of specific service rates is that they permit the costs of similar services to be compared across hospitals. This might encourage patients and physicians to give costs more weight in choosing hospitals. It has also been suggested that third parties might use this information to make co-payment and deductible payments by patients dependent on the costliness of the hospitals they use.

A disadvantage of specific services rates is that hospitals charge for hundreds of services, and a detailed review of the "reasonableness" of each rate is impossible. In practice, prospective rate setting agencies and programs typically review budgeted costs, not rates. Once a hospital's budget is agreed upon, the hospital is asked to propose a rate structure that will generate just enough revenue to cover its approved budget at its expected volume (perhaps adhering to certain guidelines; for example, that rates be set such that each patient service department comes within specified parameters of breaking even). Presumably, the commission would check the hospital's financial reports at the end of the year to determine if the rates proposed by the hospital and approved by the commission did in fact generate only the allowed revenue. Despite this shortcut (i.e., elimination of reviews of hundreds of individual rates), some commissions are beginning to consider requesting that all hospitals under their jurisdiction use a considerably simplified, uniform rate structure.

IMPACT OF PROSPECTIVE RATE SETTING ON HOSPITAL OPERATION

The impact a prospective rate setting system is likely to have on hospitals depends in large part on the basis of payment used, because the incentives posed by the different payment units differ. The areas of hospital operation that might be affected by prospective reimbursement can be identified a priori by considering the factors that determine costs in hospitals. The following is proposed as a complete although general list of these cost-influencing factors.

1. Cases treated
2. Case mix
3. Length of stay
4. Intensity of service
5. Scope of service
6. Amenity level
7. Quality level
8. Efficiency
9. Input prices
10. Investment in the improvement or maintenance of human and physical resources
11. Teaching programs

It is proposed that hospitals must act through these variables in attempting to keep their costs below their prospective rates. Further, given the payment unit used by a prospective rate setting system, the changes in these areas of operation that might be expected to occur can be predicted. It should be emphasized, however, that these predictions are based on the assumption that prospective payment is the only constraint or incentive to which hospitals must respond. Clearly, other goals and pressures affect hospitals; therefore, the predictions proposed may not hold in any particular situation.

Table 1 shows the changes in the areas of operation expected to occur under the different payment units. The payment units are ordered from the most aggregate to the most specific. It is important to note that hospital revenue under the first three payment units is not directly related to output, since once the amount to be paid is set for the prospective year, it does not vary with the actual quantity of services provided in that year. Under the other three payment units, which are in effect different measures of output, hospital revenue is directly related to output.

As Table 1 shows, the total budget, departmental budgets, or capitation bases of payment discourage increases in *cases treated* and *lengths of stay* because these methods of payment do not link the amounts hospitals are paid to the number of patients admitted or days of care provided. Hospitals might attempt to admit more selectively and to discharge patients sooner to alternative facilities or to their homes. Depending on the adequacy of payment for out-of-hospital services, hospitals might develop preadmission testing, outpatient surgery, outpatient diagnostic and treatment services, and home care programs to prevent or shorten hospitalizations.

In addition to the incentive to reduce admissions and patient days, these bases of payment provide an incentive for hospitals to contain increases in per unit costs by changing the mix of patients treated and by changing the nature of the services provided them. Hospitals might admit fewer complex or serious case types, thereby shifting toward a less costly *case-mix*. Hospitals might discontinue (or delay adding) costly programs and services, thereby reducing the *scope of service* they offer. These actions tend to reinforce each other. Hospitals might also curtail the *amenity level, quality level,* and *intensity of service* they provide. An incentive exists for hospitals to improve *efficiency,* both by increasing input productivity and by shifting toward a less costly input mix. Assuming that hospitals have some buying power, an incentive exists to resist increases in *input prices*. An incentive also exists to reduce *investments in human and physical resources.* Cuts might be made in programs designed to improve employee morale and productivity and in programs designed to prevent deterioration of equipment and physical plant (although such actions would tend to increase costs in the long run). Finally, an incentive exists to curtail *teaching programs,* both because of the direct expenditures involved, and because of the indirect impact of these programs on case-mix, intensity of service, and scope of service.

The overall effect of using any of these bases of payment in a prospective rate setting system should be to discourage

TABLE 1*

Expected Changes in Hospital Performance Under Alternative Payment Units

	Areas of performance (cost-influencing variables)										
Payment Unit	**Cases Treated**	**Length of Stay**[1]	**Complexity of Case-Mix**[2]	**Intensity of Service**[1]	**Scope of Service**	**Amenity Level**	**Quality Level**	**Efficiency**	**Input Prices**	**Investment in Resources**	**Teaching Programs**
Total hospital budget	↓	↓	↓	↓	↓	↓	↓	↑	↓	↓	↓
Departmental budgets	↓	↓	↓	↓	↓	↓	↓	↑	↓	↓	↓
Family or person (capitation)	↓	↓	↓	↓	↓	↓	↓	↑	↓	↓	↓
Case or stay	↑	↓	↓	↓	↓	↓	↓	↑	↓	↓	↓
Day	↑	↑	↓	↓	↓	↓	↓	↑	↓	↓	↓
Specific services	↑	↑ [3]	↑	↑	↑	↓	↓	↑	↓	↓	↓

[1] It is assumed that intensity of service and length of stay are not substitutes (i.e., hospitals do not have to increase intensity in order to discharge patients sooner). Underlying this assumption is the belief that reductions in lengths of stay would come from the last few days of hospitalization, which are primarily convalescent.

[2] Admissions and case-mix are interrelated in that the case types that would be denied admission if admissions were reduced would be the least complex. Therefore, the case-mix of hospitalized patients that would result would include a higher proportion of more complex case types. At the same time, however, a hospital could attempt to select easier case types whenever possible.

[3] The direction of change in length of stay depends on the occupancy level. If a hospital is operating at high occupancy and has patients waiting for admission, payment on a per service basis should cause it to discharge patients sooner (reducing the average length of stay) in order to substitute patients requiring the more service-intensive first few days of hospitalization. Hospitals operating at low occupancy could both admit more patients and increase the length of stay to increase the quantity of services produced. The direction of change indicated is based on the observation that hospitals have extra or unfilled beds much of the time.

*Reprinted with minor modifications from Dowling, W. L. "Prospective Reimbursement of Hospitals." *Inquiry* 11:3 (Sept. 1974).

increases in both the quantity and cost per unit of hospital services, so that increases in aggregate costs should be slowed.

In contrast, the overall effect on aggregate costs of using any of the output-related bases of payment—cases, days, or specific services—cannot be predicted, since they simultaneously motivate hospitals (1) to increase output (both to directly increase revenue and to spread fixed costs over more units of output to reduce the average cost per unit); and (2) to contain increases in the cost per unit of output, by containing the amenity level, quality level, intensity, and scope of service provided; by increasing efficiency; and by containing input prices, investments in resources, and teaching programs.

Specifically, payment of a fixed amount per case would motivate hospitals to admit more patients, but, if possible, to admit less complex case types, to shorten stays, and to reduce the intensity and scope of services provided. Payment of a fixed amount per day would motivate hospitals to increase the days of care provided, by increasing admissions and lengths of stay, and to shift from more costly to less costly days by admitting less complex case types and by reducing the intensity and scope of services provided. Payment of fixed amounts for specific services (e.g., nursing care, laboratory tests, surgical procedures, x-rays, etc.) would motivate hospitals to provide more services by increasing admissions and lengths of stay to increase the number of patients requiring services, and by increasing the intensity of service provided. In contrast to the other payment units, hospitals might attempt to admit the more complex case types, since they need the most services.

Figure 4a and 4b contrast the incentives inherent in the output-related and non-output-related bases of payment. Figure 4a illustrates the situation of a hypothetical hospital operating under prospective per case, per day, or per specific service rates. TC_b represents the hospital's approved budgeted costs, TR_{pr} the revenue the hospital's prospective rates will generate at different volumes, m_b the agreed to operating margin, and v_b the expected volume. Since TR_{pr} depends directly on volume, an incentive exists to increase volume or at least to keep it from falling below v_b. In addition, an incentive exists to contain costs (as represented by TC_a), whatever the volume. Both actions act to increase the operating margin. Since increases in volume increase costs while cost contain-

FIGURE 4A. PROSPECTIVE PER CASE, DAY OR SPECIFIC SERVICE RATES

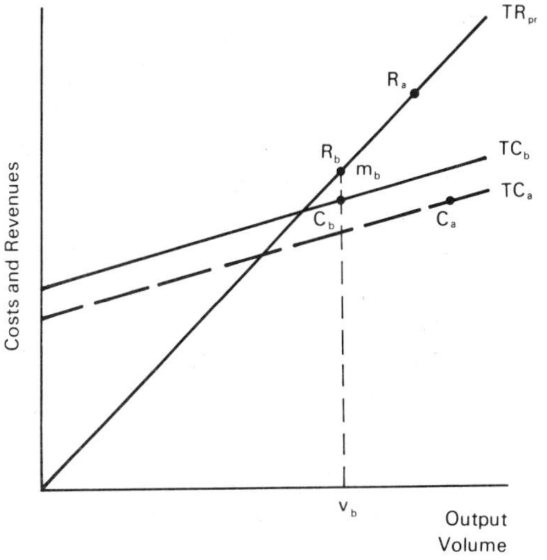

FIGURE 4B. PROSPECTIVE TOTAL BUDGET PAYMENT PROGRAM

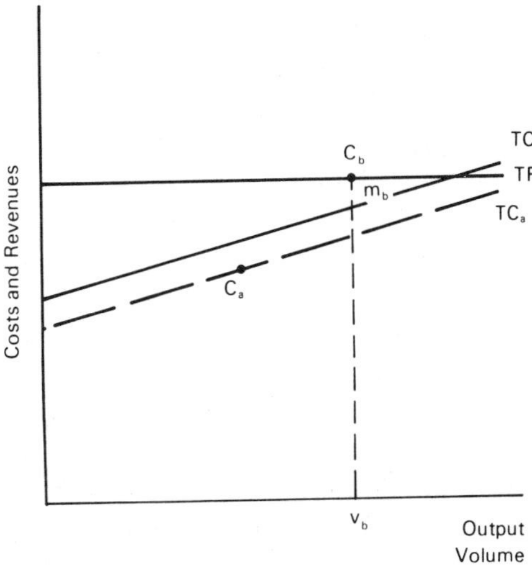

ment efforts reduce them, it cannot be predicted whether actual total costs C_a will be above or below budgeted total costs C_b. It is quite possible, however, for actual revenue R_a (which is equivalent to patient and third party outlays) to exceed budgeted revenue R_b.

Figure 4b illustrates the situation of a hypothetical hospital operating under a prospective total budget payment program. TC_b represents the hospital's approved budgeted costs and TR_{pr} its guaranteed total revenue, set so as to provide an agreed upon operating margin m_b at the expected volume v_b. Since TR_{pr} does not depend on volume, an incentive exists to reduce volume or keep it from rising above v_b. A cost containment incentive TC_a also exists. Since both actions act to reduce costs, actual total costs C_a should be below budgeted total costs C_b. It is not possible for actual revenue to exceed budgeted revenue, since the approved budget figure is all the hospital will be paid.

All of the output related payment units then provide an incentive for hospitals to increase output, and this might be reinforced by long-run goals of growth and prestige. Of concern, of course, is whether inappropriate use would result. It should be emphasized that no payment unit is without potential negative impacts, and this is a dilemma that must be faced in designing prospective rate setting systems. It appears that controls over quality and utilization may assume more importance as cost containment incentives are introduced. Another approach would be to aim additional financial incentives directly at certain areas of operation; for example, by directly rewarding hospitals for reducing their average length of stay.

The actions hospitals are likely to take under prospective rate setting systems will depend on the basis of payment used. Selection of the payment unit, therefore, depends on how one wishes to change hospital performance.

In summary, hospitals can attempt to contain costs in different ways. The actions hospitals are likely to take under prospective rate setting systems will depend on the basis of payment used. Selection of the payment unit, therefore, depends on how one wishes to change hospital performance. Hospitals could be left free to respond as best fits their situation, or additional controls could be applied to influence their responses. Hospital preferences for the different payment units would depend in part on their expectations about future use. If an increase in use is expected, the output related payment units would be preferred; if a decrease is expected, the budget or capitation payment units would be preferred. The magnitudes of the changes in operations predicted to occur under prospective rate setting depend on several factors:

1. The tightness of the prospective rates. Obviously, if hospitals must take extreme measures to maintain their financial viability, changes would be greater than if the rates were more "reasonable."
2. The firmness of the prospective rates. If rates are adjusted for actual

volume or for changes in case-mix, input prices, etc., the impact of prospective rate setting would be moderated.

3. The size of potential rewards or penalties. This depends on the proportion of any difference between actual costs and prospective rates that hospitals are at risk for and on the proportion of their patients covered by prospective payment. Also, if hospitals are able to offset potential losses by increasing charges to self pay patients, the influence of prospective rate setting would be moderated.
4. The present state of hospital performance. Admissions or lengths of stay, for example, might decrease more under the appropriate payments units in hospitals where inappropriate use is occurring than in those where there is little overuse.
5. The disposition of physicians toward cooperating with hospital cost containment efforts. Admissions, case-mix, length of stay, etc., depend largely on decisions made by physicians; and therefore, changes in the medically related areas of operation require their support.

PROSPECTIVE RATE SETTING METHODS

Prospective rate setting is a fairly recent innovation in hospital payment, and as a result, the rate setting methods currently in use are relatively unsophisticated. Although all methods attempt to establish "fair but tight" rates, the range of factors taken into account in determining rates, the degree of sensitivity to the idiosyncracies of individual institutions, the data required, and the criteria and procedures used differ greatly. In addition, the rate setting method used can affect the incentives placed on hospitals by prospective payment systems. The most commonly used rate setting methods[2] are as follows:

1. Projection of past and/or present year costs forward to become prospective year rates, with projections based upon:
   - peer group cost levels and trends,
   - economic indices,
   - normative standards,
   - or a combination of these bases.
2. Budget review to determine the reasonableness of prospective year costs and rates, with budget reviews based on:
   - comparison of budgeted costs to past year costs,
   - comparison of budgeted costs to peer group costs,
   - comparison of budgeted costs to normative cost standards,
   - or a combination of these bases.

Formulas

Negotiation is generally cited as another method of determining rates, and it is certainly conceivable that decisions about rates could depend solely upon bargaining skill and market power. However, in actual practice, negotiation tends to be the final step used to come to closure after budget reviews or projection techniques have defined a fairly narrow range of acceptable costs or rates. Whereas negotiation may serve as the final step in rate setting, "formulas" often serve as the first step. The term formula has come to mean any automatic, mechanical, rule-like method for defining acceptable parameters around costs or rates or for directly setting rates. Formulas may incorporate peer group cost means or trends, economic inflation indices, coefficients derived from statistically estimated cost functions or points derived from expert panels (both reflecting the scope and sophistication of the programs and services offered by hospitals), or simply arbitrary (or "normative") ceilings or parameters.

Formulas may be used to define how historical costs are to be projected forward into prospective rates, to translate hospital or patient characteristics into acceptable cost or rate parameters, or to define parameters that can be employed in screening budgets to identify costs that appear out of line. Generally, the application of a formula is followed by a detailed review and/or negotiation step, although in a few prospective rate-setting systems, final rates are set directly by formulas, and these rates can only be challenged by a formal appeal. Formula methods of rate setting are certainly less costly to administer than budget reviews or negotiations (although the costs of appeals and court cases may be substantial where formulas are too arbitrary or simplistic). It appears that when formulas are used to isolate questionable situations that are then considered in detail, the advantages of the cost savings inherent in formulas and the fairness and thoroughness inherent in individual reviews can both be achieved. This two-stage process has come to be called the "detailed review by exception" approach to rate setting.

Empirical Standards

Lacking normative standards of "reasonableness," empirical standards are commonly used in the budget review and projection methods of rate setting. Hospitals are grouped according to cost-influencing characteristics like ownership, location, size, scope of services, outpatient programs, teaching programs, etc. Projections or judgments about cost levels or trends can then be based on a comparison of each hospital with its peer group. Although the costs or rates for a particular hospital may appear out of line, only if the hospital is compared to truly similar hospitals can a decision that its costs are actually unreasonable be made with conviction. As a result, the characteristics considered and techniques used in grouping hospitals are critical to the effectiveness and equity of prospective rate setting. The debate between the Social Security Administration and hospital representatives about the adequacy of the grouping scheme used to establish ceilings on reasonable costs in implementing Section 223 of PL 92-603 demonstrates the concern over this matter.

Output Mix, Input Prices

Theoretically, hospitals should be grouped according to two major variables—output mix and input prices.

Output mix would be measured by the diagnostic types, complexity, and severity of patients treated by each hospital. Input prices would be measured by the price and salary levels prevailing in each hospitals' input market. Capital and teaching costs would be isolated and evaluated separately. Focusing on operating costs then, if output mix and input prices could be measured accurately enough that hospitals treating equally complex case mixes and operating in equally costly input markets could be grouped together, ceilings or projections of costs or rates based on peer group means would be defensible on the grounds that out-of-line costs could only be due to more costly than typical treatment patterns or to inefficient operations. The burden of proof would shift to high-cost hospitals to demonstrate why they could not treat a case mix of the same complexity as cheaply as the other hospitals in their peer group. However, the case mix data required to implement such a grouping scheme are not available from most hospitals, and therefore, existing grouping schemes use hospital size, services, and other structural variables instead. Although these schemes may give groupings of hospitals with fairly comparable cost structures, they do not allow the burden of proof to be shifted to high-cost hospitals as would groupings based on output mix and input prices.

PROJECTION METHODS

Projection methods of rate setting begin with a hospital's costs for the past and/or present year and extrapolate or trend them forward to become prospective year rates using group means or trends, economic indices, normative standards, or a combination of these, as bases for the projections. The New York Blue Cross formula for setting prospective rates provides an example:

Audited base year per diem cost* + % increase in estimated current year cost over base year cost** + % increase for projected input cost increases*** = Prospective per diem rate for coming year

*Adjusted downward if the hospital's average per diem cost is more than 15% above the weighted average per diem cost for its group.

**Adjusted downward (upward) if the percent increase in the hospital's per diem cost is more than 10% above (below) the percent increase in the weighted average per diem cost for its group.

***Based on a projection of the three-year moving average increase in economic indices reflecting the components of hospital costs.

This formula was used by New York Blue Cross from 1970 through 1975. Although Blue Cross has not changed its basic approach to rate setting since then, two specific changes have been made in the way in which the formula is applied that are extremely significant. First, base year cost ceilings are applied to ancillary and routine service costs separately, and second, for each, the 50th percentile average per diem cost for a hospital's peer group is used as the acceptable cost ceiling. Thus, a hospital's base year average per diem ancillary cost and its average per diem routine cost must both be at or below the 50th percentile figure for its group for formula application purposes. Note that this formula uses both peer group costs and an economic index in projecting prospective rates. The adjustments or ceilings are intended to assure that high-cost hospitals (i.e., hospitals with high base year costs or high base to intermediate year cost increases rates compared to their peers) are not automatically rewarded by high rates, and the economic index is intended to keep hospital cost increases in line with inflation rates in the general economy–an explicit goal of the New York scheme.

The best example of projections based on normative standards come from the ESP program. Phases II and III limited hospital cost and price increases to 6%, and the proposed Phase IV would have limited annual revenue per admission increases to 7.5%. Although clearly somewhat arbitrary, these figures were supposedly based on expert judgment about what was reasonable. The 7.5% figure, for example, represented a composite of (1) an estimated inflation rate of 5.9%, (2) an allowance for increased intensity of 2.5%, and (3) an adjustment or offset for improved productivity of −1.0%.

Problems

Two fundamental problems with projection methods of rate setting are apparent: (1) changes from year to year in each hospital's case mix, intensity, programs and services, etc., are not fully accounted for, and (2) long-run cost containment incentives are poor.

Since the actual costs of each hospital in the past and/or present year serve as the starting point for determining prospective year rates when projection methods are used, differences between hospitals existing initially are presumably taken into account. The problem is with changes over time. Major changes in facilities, teaching programs, or other factors used as classification variables might result in hospitals being regrouped. However, most year to year changes, unless very substantial, would not automatically be recognized in this manner. As a result, hospitals caring for a more complex case mix, for example, requiring more intensive and sophisticated services, might be penalized by inappropriately tight rates. So might a hospital adding to or upgrading its programs and services to keep up with advances in medical technology or new community needs.

To deal with these problems, grouping schemes can be refined to take more factors into account. Processes can be established for requesting rate adjustments for approved new facilities and services. A "costliness of case mix" index, as proposed in Phase IV, could be developed to show the cost implications of changes in case mix. A "costliness of services" index could be used in the same way. Diagnostic-specific per case rates might be paid, so that changes in case mix automatically influence the amounts hospitals received. Finally, an appeals process is generally available for hospitals that feel they have been treated unfairly. Nevertheless, projection methods of rate setting tend to be more arbitrary and insensitive to institutional uniquenesses than budget review methods.

When prospective rates are insensitive to changes over time in cost influencing factors like case mix, intensity, programs and services, etc., hospitals may be unfairly under or over paid. On the other hand, if changes in these factors are automatically and fully adjusted in hospital rates, the incentives deliberately imposed by prospective rate setting systems to encourage hospitals to be aware of, concerned about, and to attempt to control costs in all areas of operation are moderated. For example, many believe that prospective rate setting should encourage hospitals not only to improve their operating efficiency, but also:

1. to make definite decisions about what case types to treat and what case types to refer to other hospitals,
2. to attempt to control overuse of ancillary services and overly long lengths of stay,
3. to make cost-effective decisions about adding new programs and services,
4. to avoid duplicating services available in nearby hospitals,
5. to attempt to develop outpatient services as a substitute for inpatient care.

Those who would like to put hospitals at risk for making (or not making) cost-influencing decisions like these are reluctant to see rates adjusted too readily for actual experience during the prospective years, arguing that this eases the pressure on hospitals to act on these matters.

Another problem with projecting historical costs forward into prospective rates is that each hospital's future rates depend on its present cost containment successes. Thus, if a hospital cuts its costs one year, its rates will be lower in future years when the first year's costs become the base or starting point for rate projections. Hospitals are motivated, therefore, to spend right up to their prospective rate each year to avoid putting themselves in a tighter financial position in future years. This problem, perhaps more than anything else, has plagued the design of prospective rate setting systems. It can only be solved if rate projections are based on something other than a hospital's own cost performance. Peer group performance or normative measures of performance are possibilities. It is crucial that this problem be dealt with in the design of prospective rate setting systems, so that they truly offer positive long-run cost containment incentives, and so that efficient hospitals are rewarded and inefficient hospitals penalized.

Hospitals are motivated to spend right up to their prospective rate each year to avoid putting themselves in a tighter financial position in future years. This problem has plagued the design of prospective rate setting systems.

BUDGET REVIEW METHODS

The budget review approach to rate setting is clearly more sensitive than projection methods to differences among hospitals in the quantity and types of patients treated, facilities and services, input prices, teaching programs, amenity, quality, productivity, etc. Assuming arbitrary decision rules are not used, budget review is the fairest (in the sense of examining each hospital's situation individually) method of determining the reasonableness of costs in that it permits the affect of each cost influencing factor on each hospital to be taken into account. Hospitals have an opportunity to explain and defend their budgets, and the rate setting agency or program has an opportunity to question items that appear out of line. Budget review gives the agency more of a chance to influence specific hospital activities and plans before decisions about them are implemented.

Cost Examination

In short, a detailed, institution by institution examination of costs and cost-influencing factors characterizes the budget review method of rate setting. To many, this is the attractive feature of this method; to others, its basic drawback. Meaningful budget reviews require considerable expertise—in accounting, economics, finance, and hospital management—which many rate setting agencies and programs do not have. Comprehensive and thorough reviews also require comparable and fairly detailed cost and statistical data; a knowledge of the assumptions, modes of operation, and plans that underlie the figures presented; a knowledge of the need for new programs and services proposed; etc. The tendency is for the agency to ask for more and more data and get more and more involved. For example, suppose a hospital's radiology cost per case or per day appears high. This could be due to a case mix requiring extensive and sophisticated radiology procedures, or to the intensity of x-ray services provided to patients generally, productivity, salaries, etc., as the following formula indicates:

$$\frac{\text{Average X-Ray Cost}}{\text{Case}} = \sum \begin{array}{cccc} \underline{\textit{Case Mix}} & \underline{\textit{Intensity}} & \underline{\textit{Productivity}} & \underline{\textit{Salaries}} \\ \text{Cases}_1 \cdot & \dfrac{\text{Ave X-rays}}{\text{Case}_1} \cdot & \dfrac{\text{Ave Manhours}}{\text{X-ray}} \cdot & \dfrac{\text{Ave Salary}}{\text{Manhour}} \\ \text{Cases}_2 \cdot & \dfrac{\text{Ave X-rays}}{\text{Case}_2} \cdot & \dfrac{\text{Ave Manhours}}{\text{X-ray}} \cdot & \dfrac{\text{Ave Salary}}{\text{Manhour}} \\ \vdots & & & \end{array}$$

Questions could also be asked about the kinds of radiology procedures commonly done for each case type, the skill mix of the department's personnel, the quantity and types of supplies used, and so on. The point is, of course, that it is difficult to draw the line on "second guessing" hospital management. Few people believe that rate setting agencies can run the hospitals they are supposed to regulate as well as the governing boards and management staffs of these hospitals (typically, the management staffs of a few large hospitals taken together are larger than the entire agency staff), but it is not clear how encroachment on management prerogatives can be prevented.

Case Mix Data Approach

One approach, suggested above, is to concentrate on better case mix data rather than better operating data, so that the "burden of proof" can be shifted to hospitals whose costs appear out of line to demonstrate why they are unable to care for a case mix of comparable complexity as cheaply as their peers. Whether because of intensity, productivity, salaries, skill mix, or supplies, it would be up to the hospital to determine and correct its problems. Another more common approach is the "detailed review by exceptions" process, also discussed above, wherein budgets are screened, perhaps automatically by a computerized process, and only the third or so that appear out of line in terms of certain guidelines, parameters, or standards "flagged" for a detailed review. Thus, an administrator would know that if his budget was kept within reasonable bounds, he would not be second guessed. This concept could be furthered if the guidelines used for screening were made known in advance. An administrator could budget with these guidelines in mind, knowing that his budget would definitely not be reviewed as long as it fell within the guidelines. Finally, it should be noted that the entire process of reviewing individual hospital budgets may take place within the constraint of a predetermined aggregate state-wide cost increase limit—a "maxi-cap"—as is the case in Rhode Island.

Level of Detail

Related to this is the question of what level of detail to focus on. For example, if a hospital's "bottom line," as represented by, say, its overall cost per case compares favorably with its peers, is further review required? If so, what if its overall routine daily services cost, ancillary services cost, and "hotel" services costs are all in line, is further review required? Should reviews stop at function or program costs, departmental costs, or line item costs? Obviously, a balance between the detail of reviews and the time, effort, data requirements, etc., of carrying them out must be maintained.

Data and Staff Requirements

Two other concerns with regard to budget reviews should be mentioned. First, this approach to rate setting almost inevitably leads rate setting agencies to want hospitals to convert to a uniform chart of accounts, uniform output and productivity statistics, uniform budgeting, and uniform financial reporting, so that finer and finer comparisons can be made. Second, the budget review approach requires more and better staff than projection methods of rate setting (some estimates are as high as one budget reviewer—knowledgeable about both accounting and hospital management—for every ten hospitals), although staff requirements can be moderated somewhat by the use of screening techniques. Rate setting agencies frequently find it difficult to get an adequate budget from the state and to attract sufficient numbers of qualified personnel.

YEAR END COMPLIANCE

Compliance Check

It appears that an end-of-year "compliance check" process of some sort will become more common in prospective rate setting systems for three reasons: (1) As noted above, it is literally impossible for a rate setting agency to individually review and approve all of the

Rate setting agencies frequently find it difficult to get an adequate budget from the state and to attract sufficient numbers of qualified personnel.

rates that characterize a typical hospital's rate structure. Rather, after approving a hospital's budget for the prospective year, an agency may simply ask the hospital to propose a set of rates that in its judgment will generate just enough revenue to cover its approved costs at its expected volume. These rates are rarely reviewed in detail, and so a check may be necessary to assure that the rates are not too high. (2) Also, as noted above, per case, per day, and per specific services prospective payment systems tend to encourage hospitals to increase volume, because this acts to increase their operating margins. Hence, a check may be necessary to assure that unreasonable margins are not made as a result of increases in volume (or by deliberately underestimating volume in the budget). (3) A check may also be necessary in attempting to assure that efficient hospitals are rewarded and inefficient hospitals penalized by the prospective payment system.

Goals

The goals of an end-of-year compliance check can be examined by means of the cost-revenue-volume model. Suppose a prospective rate setting system has determined as a matter of policy that well-run hospitals should receive a certain margin above operating costs. The rate setting agency reviews and approves (perhaps after modification) hospital

FIGURE 5

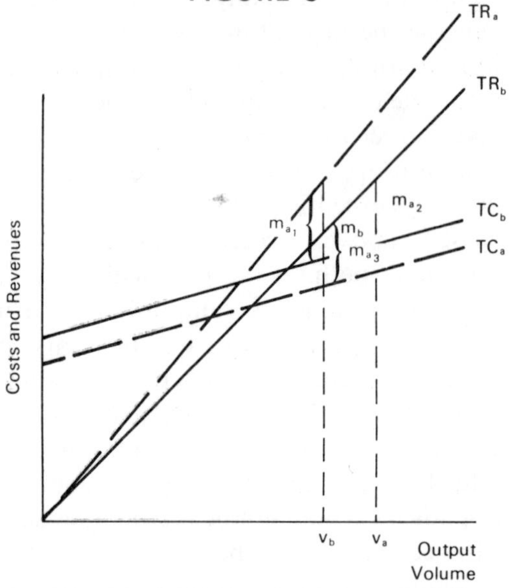

budgets and then essentially accepts the set of specific services rates proposed by each hospital as sufficient to generate just enough revenue to cover its approved costs. Figure 5 illustrates this situation. Approved budgeted cost is represented by TC_b, the revenue the approved rates will generate at different volumes by TR_b, the agreed to operating margin by m_b, and the expected volume by v_b.

Operating Margin

The actual operating margin for the prospective year may exceed the agreed to margin m_b for three reasons: (1) The rates proposed by the hospital and approved by the agency may have been "too high" as represented by TR_a (i.e., they may have generated more revenue than necessary to cover approved costs and provide the agreed to operating margin). This is shown by margin m_{a1}. Presumably, the hospital should not benefit financially from the fact that its rates were set "too high." (2) The actual volume for the year may have exceeded budgeted volume, resulting in margin m_{a2}. Presumably, the hospital should not benefit from the fact that its actual volume was higher than its budgeted volume. (3) The actual costs for the year may have been lower than budgeted costs, as reflected by TC_{a3} resulting in margin m_{a3}. Assuming that the agency's budget review was rigorous and thorough, the additional operating margin achieved in this situation can be attributed to improved operating efficiency, and presumably the hospital should benefit from its cost-containment success. In short, it appears that rate setting agencies will begin to develop methods for determining the nature of the surpluses (or losses) that hospitals experience under prospective payment in an attempt to control the system and to make sure that only deserving hospitals are rewarded by it.

POTENTIAL

As this discussion of the dilemmas and problems inherent in translating the concept of prospective rate setting into practice should make clear, prospective payment is not a simple panacea for the cost inflation problem confronting the nation's hospitals. It is not a fully developed, tested, and proven strategy, and much refinement of data, methods, and techniques will be necessary before fair but tight rates can be set with assurance. Moreover, even with refinement, few believe that rate setting, in isolation from controls over facilities, services, and utilization and mechanisms for encouraging consumers and physicians to use hospitals more prudently, can impact significantly on the cost problem.

Despite the problems, however, prospective rate setting appears to have considerable potential. Living under a fixed budget or rate is just fundamentally different from operating under the conventional methods of reimbursement. Prospective rate setting causes costs to be given more weight in decisions about current operations or future programs. It should lead to better budgeting, planning, cost finding, and cost control. It should make cash flow and revenue more predictable. It may provide a basis for straightening out differences in payment among the different third parties. Perhaps most important, it gives administrators and financial managers a clear mandate to attack the cost problem in their institutions. The critical question is whether the cost containment potential of prospective rate setting can be exploited with enough sensitivity that the quality and financial viability of the hospital system is maintained.

REFERENCES

1. Although the concepts and issues surrounding prospective rate setting appear applicable to all institutional providers, in actual practice almost all of the operating systems focus on hospitals. Hence, reference is made hereafter to "hospitals" rather than to "providers."

2. Two additional methods of rate setting have been suggested but not tried:

Determination of reasonable costs of specific services

The National Advisory Committee on Health Manpower recommended that payment of hospitals be based on:

> . . . a small number of well-defined services or treatments. Those chosen should be well enough defined so that there would be reasonable assurance of meeting the criterion of equal payment for equal services, e.g., certain laboratory or radiology procedures, or the treatment of specified orthopedic or surgical cases. Careful studies would be made to determine the reasonable cost of providing each service. Evaluation would be made of the quality of each service in the participating hospitals. For each one, all hospitals in a locality would receive an equal base payment plus an increment that varied with the standard of service.

See: National Advisory Commission on Health Manpower. *Report,* Vol. 1 (Washington, D.C.: GPO, 1967) p. 59.

Bidding

The bidding method of rate setting might operate as follows: Hospitals would submit bids reflecting their expected costs of producing specific services (for which specifications would be developed), or their expected costs per day. For each service the average of the bids would be accepted as the reasonable cost. If a hospital's actual cost per unit of service was below its bid, it would be paid its actual cost plus a varying percent of the difference between its actual cost and its bid, the percent depending on how far the hospital's bid was below the average of all bids (to encourage hospitals to make low bids). Hospitals with actual costs above their bid or above the average of the bids would suffer losses.

See: Hinderer, H., "Reimbursement: Past, Present, and Future," *Public Control and Hospital Operations,* Graduate Program in Hospital Administration, University of Chicago, 1972, pp. 4–9.

SUGGESTED READING

For more complete discussions of the great variety of possible approaches to prospective rate setting, see: Bauer, K. "Hospital Rate Setting—This Way to Salvation?" In: *Hospital Cost Containment,* Zubkoff, M. and Raskin, I. (eds.), Milbank Fund, Washington, D.C., 1976 (forthcoming); Bauer, K. and Densen, P. *Some Issues in the Incentive Reimbursement Approach to Cost Containment: An Overview,* Health Care Policy Discussion Paper No. 7, Harvard Center for Community Health and Medical Care, Harvard University, 1973; Dowling, W.L. "Prospective Reimbursement of Hospitals," *Inquiry* 6:163 (September 1974); Feldstein, P. "An Analysis of Reinbursement Plans." In: *Reimbursement Incentives for Hospital and Medical Care,* SSA Research Report No. 26, Government Printing Office, Washington, D.C., 1968; Goldstrom, G. *Prospective Payment to Hospitals: Methods of Rate Determination,* Occasional Papers in Hospital and Health Administration 2, Graduate Program in Hospital Administration, University of California, Berkeley, 1973; Hardwick, C.; Meyers, S.; and Woodruff, L. *Incentive Reimbursement: Prospects, Proposals, Plans, and Programs,* Research Series No. 6, Blue Cross of Western Pennsylvania, 1969; Laudicina, S. *Prospective Reimbursement for Hospitals: A Guide for Policymakers,* Community Service Society of New York, New York, October 1976; Pauly, M. "Efficiency, Incentives, and Reimbursement for Health Care," *Inquiry* 7:14 (March 1970); Sattler, F.L. (ed.) *Hospital Prospective Payment—Issues and Experiences,* Interstudy, Minneapolis, Minnesota, June 1976; Sigmond, R. "The Notion of Hospital Incentives," *Hospital Progress* 50:63 (January 1969); and *Prospective Reimbursement Studies, Experiments, and Demonstrations.* Social Security Administration, U.S. Department of Health, Education, and Welfare, Report to the Congress of the United States, August 1974.

Detailed descriptions of specific prospective rate setting systems can be found in:

Arthur D. Little—

The Prospective Reimbursement Program of Connecticut Blue Cross, Office of Research and Statistics, Social Security Administration, 1974.

The Prospective Reimbursement Programs in the State of Colorado, Office of Research and Statistics, Social Security Administration, 1974.

The Prospective Reimbursement Program of Blue Cross

of Northeast Pennsylvania, Office of Research and Statistics, Social Security Administration, 1974.

The Prospective Hospital Rate Review Program for Blue Cross of Wisconsin Payments to Hospitals. Office of Research and Statistics, Social Security Administration, 1974.

The Prospective Reimbursement Program of Blue Cross of Northeast Ohio, Office of Research and Statistics, Social Security Administration, 1974.

The Prospective Reimbursement Program of Blue Cross of Northeast Ohio, Office of Research and Statistics, Social Security Administration, 1974.

Bauer, Katharine G.—

The Combined Budget Review and Formula Approach to Prospective Reimbursement by the Blue Cross of Western Pennsylvania. Harvard Center for Community Health and Medical Care, April, 1974.

Bauer, Katharine G. and Clark, Arva R.—

The New Jersey Budget Review Program. Harvard Center for Community Health and Medical Care, March, 1974.

The Indiana Controlled Charges System. Harvard Center for Community Health and Medical Care, March, 1974.

Budget Reviews and Prospective Rate Setting for Rhode Island Hospitals. Harvard Center for Community Health and Medical Care, February, 1974.

New York: The Formula Approach to Prospective Reimbursement. Harvard Center for Community Health and Medical Care, March 1974.

2

Prospective Rate Setting in Rhode Island

Armand P. Leco

Topics in this chapter include:

CHALLENGING THE SYSTEM
PROGRAM OVERVIEW
MAJOR PROVISIONS OF THE PROGRAM
RESPONSIBILITIES OF THE PARTIES
THE PROGRAM EXPERIENCE

WITHIN THE LAST several years, there has been an intensified interest and concern in the rising costs of health care in this country, particularly since those costs continue to outpace the rest of the economy. The Federal government has recently attempted to confront the health care cost spiral through coordination of health planning and, more recently, the implementation of cost controls or limits through Federal health care programs such as Medicare. In addition, state and local communities have been encouraged by the Federal government to apply cost control measures to the health care industry. In an equally concerned response, some state governments have established rate setting commissions to review and approve hospital rates. Among these are Connecticut, New Jersey, Massachusetts, and Maryland. At the same time, the voluntary sector, notably the Blue Cross plans, have implemented and are implementing cost containment programs to curb the growth of hospital costs. Cost containment has also been constantly espoused by the Blue Cross Association, as well as by the American Hospital Association. These approaches to cost containment are varied and are being met with varied degrees of success. However, one fact is clear—appropriate methods to moderate and contain health care costs in this country must be found.

One fact is clear—appropriate methods to moderate and contain health care costs in this country must be found. Our health care resources are no longer limitless even though the demand for health care services continues to grow.

Our health care resources are no longer limitless even though the demand for health care services continues to grow. Finally, the health care system, as well as other segments of our economy, e.g. energy, education, is finding itself in the classic economic dilemma of trying to meet those growing and seemingly un-

This article was based on work performed pursuant to Contract Number 600-75-1045 with the Social Security Administration, Department of Health, Education and Welfare.

limited demands within the confines of limited resources.

In Rhode Island, Blue Cross, all voluntary hospitals, and the State have taken action to confront this problem in a voluntary, non-regulatory setting. In 1971, this community embarked on a prospective reimbursement program, abandoning the old retrospective cost reimbursement system. This program has gone through several major changes since 1971; and, under a contract from the Social Security Administration, Blue Cross, the State, and all sixteen voluntary hospitals are entering the third year of a prospective reimbursement experiment. The following will describe that system in Rhode Island, the responsibilities of its participants, and the experience to date.

CHALLENGING THE SYSTEM

Prospective Reimbursement in Rhode Island came at the heels of three years of soaring health care demands and costs in the State. Like the rest of the nation, Rhode Island faced increased demand for hospital services, as well as a sharp increase in hospital costs with the introduction of Medicare. Combined with this was the fact that Medicare temporarily reduced the elderly's drain on Blue Cross reserves; and, taking advantage of this situation, Blue Cross of Rhode Island was able to upgrade the benefits in its subscriber contract. The result was increased demand by Blue Cross subscribers for hospital care. These two factors, increased demand and rising costs, quickly forced Blue Cross of Rhode Island to seek substantial rate increases for three consecutive years. During hearings on the third year's requested rate increase, the State's Director of Business Regulation, who regulates Blue Cross rates in Rhode Island, challenged the existing reimbursement system. He blamed the cost pass-through mechanism of the retrospective cost reimbursement contract between Blue Cross and Rhode Island hospitals as the major factor in the cost spiral. He essentially "ordered" the parties to overhaul the reimbursement system to include some form of cost ceilings and savings incentives.

Response to the Challenge

Blue Cross of Rhode Island (Blue Cross), the State's sixteen voluntary hospitals, and the Hospital Association of Rhode Island (HARI) responded and took the initiative to design and implement a "prospective reimbursement" program with the following features:

1. For FY 1970/71, Rhode Island Hospital, the largest hospital in the State, suggested to Blue Cross its willingness to negotiate its budget. This later served as a pilot for the program. All other hospitals agreed to reduce their budget requests and "guaranteed" the budgets for the fiscal year. The results of this first year showed aggregate hospital gross operating expenses being under budget for the first time ever. It was also the first time that some institutions operated with a budget.
2. In FY 1971/72, all hospitals submitted their budget requests to

Blue Cross for review and a line-by-line analysis of salaries and wages, supplies and expenses, depreciation and interest, and new programs. Final budget settlements were reached through negotiations between the parties. It is worth noting that the second year of the program resulted in negotiated settlements of only 13 percent.

3. The negotiated budgets were submitted to a cost finding process and from this, hospital rates were established.
4. Volume parameters were provided to essentially protect hospitals from unexpected volume.
5. Incentives were incorporated into the program in that hospitals absorbed 100 percent of all losses; while revenue gains were shared with Blue Cross on a 50/50 basis.
6. A unique provision incorporated area wide planning; and, hospitals agreed to defer, alter, or abandon programs that did not receive the approval of a medical program review mechanism.

In July 1971, the Rhode Island General Assembly involved the State in the process by passing legislation that made the State Budget Office a party to budget negotiations with the hospitals and Blue Cross. Prior to this, the State's only "budget control" had essentially been limited to indirect control through the Department of Business Regulation's approval or disapproval of Blue Cross rates. With the State's entrance into the program there were essentially three participants to the program: hospitals, the State, and Blue Cross. A close relationship quickly developed between Blue Cross and the State, who collectively represented approximately 90 percent of hospital business, in dealing with the hospitals.

ESP

Up until FY 1972/73, Rhode Island received a waiver from the Economic Stabilization Program (ESP) which allowed it to operate under the Prospective Reimbursement Program. However, when ESP entered Phase III, it was realized that the prospective reimbursement program was not consistent with ESP controls, and the program was suspended. All the parties agreed to develop and submit a revised prospective reimbursement program that would qualify for an exemption under ESP.

Before the parties could receive an exemption from the Cost of Living Council, the Economic Stabilization Program ended on April 30, 1974. However, work had already been completed to begin implementation of a new prospective reimbursement program in Rhode Island. And, for FY 1974/75 the parties again embarked on a cost containment program for the State. Subsequent to negotiations with the Social Security Administration, Rhode Island's prospective reimbursement program received a contract under Sec. 222 of P. L. 92-603 for a three-year experiment in cost containment and a waiver of the Medicare cost limitations under Sec. 223. The experimental contract began October 1, 1974 and extends to September 30, 1977. The present program has now entered its third year.

The following is a description of that program.

PROGRAM OVERVIEW

Like the earlier prospective reimbursement program, the present program's participants are Blue Cross of Rhode Island, the Budget Office of the State of Rhode Island, the Hospital Association of Rhode Island, and the Association's participating sixteen voluntary hospitals. Blue Cross, which represents both its own subscribers and the Social Security Administration as Medicare intermediary in Rhode Island, is the program administrator. The State Budget Office represents the State's interests as purchasers of health care through Medicaid, Title V, the Department of Vocational and Rehabilitative Services and General Public Assistance, as well as the interests of the general population of Rhode Island. The parties are operating under a three-year contract between the sixteen hospitals and Blue Cross, as an amendment to the basic hospital contract, for fifteen participating hospitals and a separate contract with the one non-participating institution, and a separate contract between each hospital and the State. It is interesting and significant to note that these contracts are only about to be signed and that the participants have voluntarily entered the program under the terms of the Prospective Reimbursement Protocol which was jointly submitted by the participants to the Social Security Administration under the experiment provisions of Sec. 222 of PL 92-603.

Social Security Administration

The Social Security Administration has been mentioned several times. Their participation in the program is both direct and indirect under the terms of the prospective reimbursement experiment contract. The Office of Research and Statistics (SSA) has the responsibility for monitoring and administering prospective reimbursement experiments under Sec. 222 of PL 92-603. And, although ORS keeps in constant contact with the program and has provided technical assistance, they have chosen to maintain a low profile in the experiment (except for direct participation in the development of the MAXICAP) and give the voluntary program an opportunity to function.

Basic Objectives

The program's basic objectives are:

1. Contain costs;
2. Assure growth in programs is based on statewide need;
3. Shift health resources from inpatient care modalities;
4. Reward management efficiencies and improve productivity;
5. And, ensure that cost control efforts do not have a deleterious effect on patient care.

Basic Features

And the basic features of the present program include:

1. A limit on total allowable operating expense increases on a statewide basis (a MAXICAP).

2. Submission of new and expanded medical programs to a planning, review, and advisory process *prior* to budget negotiations. Capital programs must also be reviewed under the State's certificate of need legislation.
3. After internal review and analysis by Blue Cross and the State Budget Office, each hospital budget (both total expenses and statistical volumes) is then negotiated with that hospital. The participants in that budget negotiation are Blue Cross, the State Budget Office and the affected hospital. The Social Security Administration may have a representative present as an observer. HARI, in addition to being present as an observer, may also provide technical assistance to the hospital.
4. Rates are set on the basis of the ratio of lower of costs or charges and according to each third party payer's reimbursement principles, after the budget has been negotiated and the final budget has been submitted to cost finding. Hospitals also agree to guarantee their charge structure as determined for the budget fiscal year.
5. Provisions are made to reimburse the hospitals for any unusual and unexpected increases in volume that may occur, as well as other major unforeseen and unpredictable expenses (major contingencies).

All of this activity is aimed at controlling the overall increases in hospital costs and yet provide sufficient flexibility within the overall dollar controls to permit hospitals to utilize their dollars to provide planned services and programs and improve the quality of care to their patients. Also, hospitals are provided incentives for management efficiencies and improved productivity. On a broader, statewide scale, the program is designed to contain the growing cost spiral of health care in Rhode Island and provide an effective, rational method of allocating and redistributing the State's ever diminishing health care resources to meet the ever growing needs and demands of the community. Above all, it has been and is still the intent of all the program participants to do this within the voluntary sector and demonstrate that given a well designed program and the proper tools the voluntary sector can control itself.

This has been a simple overview of the Rhode Island program. The specifics of how that program works, the responsibilities it places on its participants, and the experience of the last two years of the program are outlined in the following sections.

MAJOR PROVISIONS OF THE PROGRAM

Statewide MAXICAP

The most significant feature of the Rhode Island Program is the statewide MAXICAP. The MAXICAP is an outside guarantee on the aggregate gross operating expenses of the voluntary hospitals in Rhode Island for a fiscal year,

Above all, it has been and is still the intent of all the program participants to do this within the voluntary sector and demonstrate that given a well designed program and the proper tools the voluntary sector can control itself.

excluding expenses associated with professional components (i.e. Medicare, Part B) and activities financed by grants and contracts. These latter two categories of expenses are not directly controlled under the program. It must be stressed that the MAXICAP is not a target for expenses, but is a ceiling or outside limitation within which all hospital budgets must be negotiated and a reserve maintained for unforeseen expenses during the fiscal year. This does not mean that each hospital is given an across-the-board increase equal to the MAXICAP. The parties are free to negotiate hospital budgets above or below the limit of the CAP. However, in the aggregate when budget negotiations are complete, the MAXICAP shall not be exceeded. The goal is to maintain a ceiling on total expenses while providing the flexibility to recognize problems, programmatic development, unusual circumstances, etc. at a given institution.

Each spring, prior to the beginning of the next fiscal year and individual hospital budget negotiations, a committee of representatives of Blue Cross, the State, and HARI (representing its sixteen member hospitals) meets to negotiate the MAXICAP. While the Social Security Administration may be present as an observer to these negotiations, it directly participates as a third party in the development of the MAXICAP position, including initial and final percentages.

DEVELOPING POSITIONS

Blue Cross, the State and HARI each develop their MAXICAP positions prior to negotiations. This is done by first weighting the budgetary components of a hospital's budget, i.e. salaries and wages represent approximately 55–65 percent of a hospital's gross operating expenses. Then using the historical experience of hospitals, economic trends, both national and local, as may be reflected in such indices as the consumer price index and the wholesale price index; the labor contract experience, both nationally and locally; economists' predictions for the upcoming fiscal year; rates of interest; anticipated or known Federal, State, and local regulations which may impact expenses; known medical and capital programmatic development that has been approved by the planning process; and, any other relevant factors that may have a bearing on hospital operating costs, the parties mutually develop and negotiate inflation or growth factors which are then applied to the budgetary components. The result is a tabulation of percentage increases for salaries and wages, physician salaries and fees, supplies and expenses, depreciation and interest, the carryover effect of new and expanded programs implemented in the prior year, new programs, volume and intensity, etc. The sum of these factors plus a reserve factor for unforeseen expenses and volume/intensity fluctuations equals a MAXICAP percentage increase for the next fiscal year. The resulting MAXICAP is a negotiated compromise of the parties' initial positions. This final percentage is then multiplied by the current fiscal year's expense base (negotiated expense budgets plus allowances for volume, patient mix, and major contingencies) to arrive at a "pot of dollars" to be distributed among the sixteen voluntary hospitals based on the results of individual hospital budget negotiations. Examples of this process have been:

FY 1974–75	13.85%	or	approximately $193M
FY 1975–76	11.5%	or	approximately $216M
FY 1976–77	10.5%	or	approximately $238M

It is intended that the MAXICAP will not be exceeded during the fiscal year. However, there will always be unforeseen expenses due to unexpected volume expenses, extraordinary unforeseen expenses such as the significant increase in malpractice insurance premiums, etc. The reserve factor in the MAXICAP was designed to absorb such expenses. There may, however, be occasions when the reserve is insufficient for that purpose. In these instances the MAXICAP may be exceeded by mutual agreement of the program participants. This will be addressed later.

Control of hospital costs and the rational distribution of resources to meet the demands of the health care community cannot fully take place unless planning is linked to the reimbursement system.

Program Planning

Another important aspect, perhaps the first of its kind, of the Rhode Island program is the integration of health care planning with the reimbursement function. Control of hospital costs and the rational distribution of resources to meet the demands of the health care community cannot fully take place unless planning is linked to the reimbursement system. Recent passage of PL 93-641 has acknowledged this fact. In Rhode Island, both the review and approval of capital projects and the review of new and/or expanded medical programs are linked to the prospective reimbursement program.

REVIEW AND APPROVAL

Rhode Island has for some time had a review mechanism for certificate of need. All major capital projects that meet the dollar threshold are submitted to the Rhode Island Department of Health for review. Only those projects receiving the Department's approval are given consideration during budget negotiations with the costs of interest, depreciation, and general operating expenses subject to the same scrutiny and negotiations as any other budget item.

In addition, there is a unique mechanism for review of medically oriented programs. This review process was part of the original prospective reimbursement program in 1971 and was again incorporated in the revised program. Each spring, hospitals are required, under the terms of the Blue Cross Member Hospital Contract, to submit those new and/or expanded medically oriented programs that meet a predetermined dollar threshold[1] to the voluntary Health Planning Council (HPC) for review. HPC then reviews and evaluates those program requests based on a predetermined set of criteria relating to proof of community need, consistency with the hospital's goals and objectives, relationship to other community programs, consideration of appropriate alternatives, the scope of the program, programmatic costs, and program effectiveness. Based on its findings, HPC then ranks the programs and assigns priorities: Priority I—those programs that should be implemented within the fiscal year; Priority II—programs with merit that may require more planning; and, Priority III—programs which should not be implemented. HPC further prioritizes the Priority I programs. Those rankings are then transmitted to the Third Parties for consideration in budget negotiations.

Only those programs which receive a Priority I ranking are considered by the Third Parties with the program budgets and dates of implementation subject to negotiations. It must be noted that all Priority I programs may not be automatically accepted for implementation in a given fiscal year. Like any other budget item, new programs are subject to the availability of resources within the MAXICAP.

A hospital may also budget any other programs which are not specifically subject to review by HPC or the Department of Health. These programs are also subject to budget negotiations and are carefully considered where a hospital can demonstrate need and cost effectiveness. However, it must be noted that priority must be given to those programs approved by the planning process due to the limit of resources within the MAXICAP.

Hospital Budgets/Budget Negotiations

A cornerstone of the Rhode Island program is the negotiation of each hospital's budget. As previously noted, the MAXICAP provides the flexibility to settle an individual hospital's budget above or below the MAXICAP percentage. The ultimate objective is to negotiate a budget that meets the hospital's operational needs and which is justifiable from the Third Parties' point of view, while still maintaining the integrity of the MAXICAP. Several provisions are necessary for this process to be successful.

1. **The Budget Package.** Each hospital is required to submit on or about June 15 (after MAXICAP negotiations are completed) a detailed budget request for the next fiscal year. The budget submission is a twenty-two page document mutually developed and agreed to by all parties and includes detailed schedules of: a summary of revenues and expenses, salary expense, fringe benefits, physician fees and salaries, supplies and expenses, interest expense, depreciation on plant and equipment, total depreciable assets, new and expanded programs, increases due

to volume, new and expanded programs implemented in the current fiscal year, personnel/man-hours, summary of selected statistics, and narrative information explaining budgeting techniques and any unusual expenses or items for consideration. Each schedule must provide budget data for the present fiscal year, the prior year, and the budget year by major service. In addition, since all hospitals subscribe to the Commission on Professional and Hospital Activities, they are requested to furnish PAS length of stay summary data for the last twelve months. Hospitals may also submit any other additional information in support of their budget requests.

2. **IHDS Data.** Hospitals must also submit IHDS (Interagency Hospital Data Service System, a locally designed statistical reporting system) data on a monthly basis which provides statistical and financial information by individual hospital. Among the data provided is inpatient utilization by major service, including bed counts, admissions, incurred patient days, and occupancy rates; patient revenue, actual as compared to budget; paid man-hours by major department; gross operating expenses including salaries and wages, supplies and expenses, depreciation and interest, etc.; and, selected ancillary statistics by major department.

   As can be readily seen, the information provided via IHDS is very similar to that provided in the budget package. The reason for this will be evident in the discussion of budget analysis.

3. **Budget Review and Analysis.** With the necessary data available to the parties, the basis exists for rational review and analysis of a hospital's budget.

   The Third Parties' review and analysis of a hospital's budget are designed to rationally assess the hospital's needs in the budget year. The process begins with a categorization of the budget package and other relevant data:

- Identification of significant budget changes.
- Comparisons between miscellaneous revenues and expenses to actual data.
- Cost per unit of service analysis is completed, utilizing selected statistics on the basis of impact on hospital cost.
- Total operating expenses are reviewed by comparing projected actual and budgets of a prior period to current fiscal year budget.
- A quantitative analysis by bed size, unit size, and by type of hospital (i.e. teaching hospitals) is performed.
- Additionally, each major unit of service is analyzed for volume, man-hours, salaries and wages, fringes, supplies and expenses, depreciation and interest, etc.

After the above statistical information and comparisons are arrayed, each hospital's budget is analyzed in relation to national, regional and local norms reflecting: costs per unit of service, cost per type of hospital, costs per bed size, salary and wage analysis, nursing service costs per patient day, etc. At the same time, an individual hospital's productivity and performance from one year to the next is analyzed and evaluated. Additional analytical information is also obtained from such sources as Hospital Administrative Services data, the American Hospital Association's annual report, a Comparative Cost Report as compiled by Hospital Association of Rhode Island, and various positions identified during MAXICAP negotiations. All of the above are utilized to assess the reasonableness of a hospital's budget request, both on a line-by-line basis and in its entirety forming the basis for the Third Parties' position on a given hospital's budget.

However, when all is said and done with the budget package, IHDS data, and the review and analysis of each hospital's budget submission, the end result—a mutually agreed upon fiscal year budget—is reached through budget negotiations. Rather than rely on any artificially imposed budget for a hospital, either via governmental fiat or other arbitrary limitation, the parties have chosen to negotiate hospital budgets. The participants in those negotiations are the hospital, Blue Cross and the State collectively, and HARI, both to observe and to provide technical assistance to the hospital.

Initial negotiating positions center around the hospital budget submission—the hospital defending its initial request and the Third Parties presenting an initial position based on their review and analysis of the budget. From that point, budget negotiations are aimed at agreement on a total "bottomline" budget settlement (both dollars and statistics), although during the course of negotiations, each side may choose to argue specific positions on various issues, such as: salaries and wages, inflation, new programs, etc. However, within that "bottomline" settlement, the parties do identify specific dollar amounts, dates of implementation, and statistics for HPC Priority I programs and capital projects approved by the Department of Health.

The intent of the Rhode Island program is to maintain the management prerogatives of the institution to allocate its resources in the best manner possible to achieve the institution's goals.

It should be noted that negotiations are not limited to dollar amounts alone. As mentioned, the parties also negotiate the statistics associated with the budget. The importance of this aspect of the program will become evident in a later discussion on rate setting and volume.

The intent of the Rhode Island program is to maintain the management prerogatives of the institution to allocate its resources in the best manner possible to achieve the institution's goals. Therefore, the parties, while reviewing on a line-by-line basis, do not negotiate line-by-line settlements but have opted for the bottomline approach. This provides the hospital with the flexibility to manage its budget as it sees fit and its only obligations are to live within that negotiated budget and any specific agreements made on new programs. The entire goal is to leave the management and operation of Rhode Island hospitals to the institutions themselves.

Rate Determination

The establishment of rates for Rhode Island hospitals is more indirect than the approach used by a rate setting commission, for example. Primary emphasis is the negotiation of hospital expense budgets within the overall limit of a MAXICAP. Thus, rate determination is a by-product of this process. Hospital rates are established from the results of budget negotiations, budget cost finding, and the hospital's establishment of its charge structure. Since budget negotiations have already been addressed, the other two components will be briefly discussed and then all three related to the establishment of a hospital rate.

1. **Hospital Charges.** Hospitals are free to change their charges once during the fiscal year. Each hospital must determine a list of board approved hospital charges and dates of implementation at the beginning of the fiscal year. These are then transmitted to the Third Parties. Each hospital agrees to "guarantee" that charge list for the fiscal year. It may not be changed unless a hospital is granted a major contingency. In most cases, the hospital is free to establish whatever charges it feels are necessary for the institution. However, the Third Parties carefully review each charge list submitted by a hospital and will challenge the hospital on the appropriateness of those charges if increases for the upcoming fiscal year appear questionable or unreasonable.

   Given the proposed charge list and the statistics negotiated with the expense budget, the hospital then establishes its revenue budget for the fiscal year.

2. **Cost Finding.** Subsequent to negotiation of each hospital's budget, each hospital is required to process its budget through one of two computerized, simultaneous equation cost allocation systems. A single cost finding is run and adjusted for each major purchaser of care consistent with that purchaser's principles of reimbursement. For example, the cost finding for Blue Cross purposes assumes a straight-line method for depreciation; while under certain circumstances, Medicare recognizes accelerated depreciation.

   The two cost finding methods used by Rhode Island hospitals are MICAH and COSAL. MICAH is, of course, a nationally known system. COSAL is a local system, similar to MICAH, which was developed and is administered by HARICOMP, the data processing arm of HARI. Both allocation systems are recognized by Blue Cross, the State, and the Social Security Administration.

Based on the results of the cost finding process and in conjunction with the hospital's charge structure and revenue budget, ratios of allowable costs to hospital charges (RCCs) are established for each major purchaser of care based on the lower figure of costs or charges principle. Each purchaser of care has two RCCs—one for inpatient and one for outpatient. These RCCs are guaranteed prospectively by Blue Cross, the State and Medicare (SSA) and are the basis for hospital reimbursement.

In short, the Rhode Island Prospective Reimbursement program is one which indirectly establishes and regulates hospital rates, with the major emphasis being control of the major element affecting those rates—hospital operating expenses. Up to this point, the emphasis of the discussion has been the concept of the MAXICAP and how expenses, and ultimately, rates are established. The program does, however, contain two major provisions which provide exemptions to the MAXICAP; the negotiated expense budget; and, in some cases, the established prospective rates of reimbursement. These provisions are volume and patient mix and major contingencies.

Volume/Patient Mix

Volume has been a major point of controversy in the Rhode Island program. When the program was originally designed, the MAXICAP and the negotiated budget were all inclusive, including any unexpected volume that might occur. Hospitals quickly pointed out that they could not insure the risk of potential volume increases. Blue Cross and the State Budget Office conceded and established volume corridors for inpatient routine and ancillary services. There was some dispute about the intent and operation of these corridors in the first year of the program and these have subsequently been revised and a volume corridor has been added for outpatient services. However, it is generally accepted that these volume corridors are designed to protect hospitals against the costs of unexpected volume and are not financial incentives. However, the volume corridor provisions do provide an incentive for hospitals to optimally use their facilities and shift, where possible, costly inpatient care to the less expensive outpatient modalities.

The inpatient volume corridors are so designed that an institution will be reimbursed for increased or decreased volume in relation to fixed costs when activity is decreasing and variable costs when activity is increasing. There is also a volume corridor for outpatient services. However, hospitals are only reimbursed for increased outpatient volume with no adjustment for decreased volume. The key to the corridors is the hospital's budget revenue which is directly related to statistics. Since the operation of the corridors is related to statistics, this shows why, as previously noted, the negotiated budget statistics are so important to the process.

The inpatient volume corridor is divided into two categories—routine and ancillary. Days are the yardstick for measuring fluctuations in routine volume. A sliding scale adjustment to the budgeted per diem is made as actual inpatient days vary from budget days.[2] The inpatient ancillary adjustment is based on a variation of actual inpatient ancillary revenue versus budget inpatient ancillary revenue.[3] Since the revenue is the function of budgeted statistics and the hospital's charge structure, again the volume adjustment is related to a fluctuation in actual statistics versus budget statistics. As volume increases, a hospital receives only 35 percent of excess revenues generated to offset variable costs. When volume decreases, a 65 percent factor is applied to "uncollected" revenues and paid to the hospital to defray fixed costs.

The outpatient corridor functions similar to the inpatient ancillary corridor.[4] Any adjustment is based on a variation of actual revenues to budget which is a function of the outpatient budget statistics. A factor of 60 percent of excess revenues is passed on to the hospital to cover variable cost and to provide an incentive to increase outpatient modalities of care. There is no adjustment for decreased outpatient volume.

In all cases of the volume corridors, both the hospital's budgeted expenses and revenues may be affected. As volume increases, not only may the hospital retain the appropriate percentage of revenues collected but it may also adjust its budgeted expenses by a similar amount. Therefore, it can be readily seen that volume may cause a hospital to legitimately exceed its agreed upon budgeted revenues and expenses; and, in the aggregate, hospitals may exceed the MAXICAP should the reserve component of the MAXICAP be inadequate to cover the magnitude of the increased volume.

A related provision is that the program provides consideration for a possible change in patient mix. The patient mix adjustment is similar to that defined under Phase IV of ESP. However, after proving that a change in patient mix has occurred, the adjustment to negotiated expenses is negotiable between the hospital and Third Parties. The adjustment applies only to a change of patient mix requiring more intensity of care and not to a change requiring a decreased intensity. Again, as with the volume corridors, a hospital experiencing a change in patient mix may legitimately exceed its negotiated revenue and expense budgets; and, in the aggregate, hospitals may exceed the MAXICAP should the reserve factor be exceeded.

The actual impact of these provisions will be discussed later. However, as one might think, it did not result in a decrease of the aggregate expense budgets of the hospitals.

Major Contingency

The Rhode Island program also provides protection of all parties against unexpected and unforeseen events which may impact hospital expenses, such as: regulatory or statutory changes; "acts of God"; unusual increases in items like the unusual, unexpected rise in malpractice premiums two years ago; etc. Consideration for a major contingency may be requested by either the hospitals or the Third Parties, should the latter note an event which might cause a reduction in hospital expenses.

If a major contingency is granted, this again could cause a hospital to legitimately increase its budgeted revenues and expenses and, in the aggregate, may cause the MAXICAP to be exceeded should the reserve factor be exceeded. In addition, if the granting of a major contingency causes a problem whereby charges are lower than costs, a hospital may request a change in its charges and its prospective reimbursement rate may be changed.

Until now, this article has concerned itself with the major provisions of the program: the MAXICAP; health planning; hospital budgets, review, and analysis; budget negotiations; rate determination; and ways in which both the MAXICAP and negotiated budgets may be exceeded—volume/patient mix and major contingencies. Within those sections, the responsibilities of hospitals and the Third Parties have been addressed. It is, however, appropriate to capsulize those responsibilities for the reader's convenience.

RESPONSIBILITIES OF THE PARTIES

The advent of Prospective Reimbursement brought increased responsibilities of the participants, both hospitals and the Third Parties. No longer could the parties operate under the ease of a retrospective cost reimbursement system.

Hospitals' Responsibility

For hospitals, prospective reimbursement demanded increased financial responsibility and expertise, including:

- Improved budgeting techniques and forecasting ability.
- Increased financial and statistical reporting.
- Additional budget management capabilities.
- Improved management efficiencies and operational productivity.
- Increased utilization of management engineering techniques, shared services, and other cost-saving techniques.

Not only did these requirements improve the hospitals' management responsibility for its budgeted expenses and financial controls, it also provided a major incentive to the institutions. If, as a result of improved budget management, a hospital can generate savings within its negotiated budget, it is free to use those savings to further improve or expand its institutional services and programs, within the limits of the overall program.

Third Party Responsibility

As the responsibilities of hospitals increased, so did the responsibilities of the Third Parties, including:

- Management of the statewide MAXICAP.
- Improved financial expertise and forecasting abilities.
- Expanded ability for budget review, analysis and budget negotiations.
- The ability to effectively monitor hospital financial performance.
- Better integration of the planning process.

The two most important responsibilities of the Third Parties are management of the MAXICAP and monitoring of hospital financial performance. Prior to prospective reimbursement, the Third Parties' responsibility for controlling hospital expenses was limited. Under the present program, the Third Parties are

All sections of the nation's health care delivery system are questioning cost containment and cost controls.

given the responsibility to manage and allocate over $200 million to appropriately provide for the State's hospital needs and assure that the allocation is accomplished in a fair and equitable manner. Additionally, management responsibility has increased the need to be able to monitor hospital financial performance on an ongoing basis. To accomplish this, Blue Cross has developed a computerized budget monitoring system, utilizing the hospitals' financial and statistical reporting, to track hospital spending, volume, revenues, etc. during the year and identify and analyze reimbursement problems prior to the end of the fiscal year when it may be too late to correct.

All sections of the nation's health care delivery system are questioning cost containment and cost controls. Within this context it must be realized that cost containment programs increase the responsibilities of all parties. It's not only hospitals that are affected, but Third Party payer responsibilities must also increase especially in an environment that is attempting to maintain the viability of the voluntary system in cost containment.

THE PROGRAM EXPERIENCE

Since its inception in October 1974, the Prospective Reimbursement Program in Rhode Island has had its share of growing pains and problems and has been met with varied success. During each year of the experiment, the MAXICAP has been reduced. In addition, although many hospitals continue to experience some difficulty in holding their spending to their negotiated budgets, the level of hospital overspending has also decreased. It would appear that the experiment has had a positive effect on this development; however, any definitive conclusions cannot be made until the final analysis upon completion of the experiment. At the same time, the program has been modified to more adequately meet the needs and objectives of the participants and improve the program's effectiveness in cost containment.

Financial Evaluation

A full financial/statistical evaluation of the first two years is difficult since the final audited numbers are not yet available and the Third Parties have not had the opportunity to fully analyze those figures. The figures presented here are the best approximations of the results at the present time and should provide a frame of reference. For example, in FY 1974–75, Blue Cross, the State Budget Office, HARI and its sixteen member hospitals negotiated a MAXICAP of 13.85 percent. Aggregate hospital budgets, as negotiated, totaled an increase of 12.58 percent over the prior year; and, it appeared that the program was off to a strong start. However, toward the end of the first year, it became apparent that aggregate hospital spending would exceed both the aggregate negotiated budgets and the MAXICAP. The magnitude of the increase was greater than 15.2 percent over FY 1973–74. This disappointing performance in the first year was offset to some extent by the fact that the rest of the nation experienced increased costs of 17 to 18 percent. Despite this fact, the Third Parties were deeply concerned about the situation.

The Problem

There were three major causes for the problem in FY 1974–75: malpractice, losses, and volume. Malpractice expenses increased sharply in FY 1974–75; and, hospitals were granted a major contingency to cover the impact of those expenses. The program prescribes that losses, hospital expenses in excess of the agreed upon budget, and volume and major contingency adjustments be absorbed, 100 percent, by the hospitals themselves. However, the malpractice major contingency and losses, as noted, do not explain the additional 1.3 percent increase in hospital spending. This was attributable to volume and the operation of the volume corridors which led to a major disagreement between the Third Parties and the hospitals as to the operation of the original volume corridors. Hospitals considered these volume corridors as an incentive under Prospective Reimbursement. On the other hand, the Third Parties' interpretation was that the volume corridors should only operate to protect hospitals from inordinate volume increases and the expenses associated with such increases and should not be an avenue to generate excess revenues or gains. Having identified this problem, the parties met and renegotiated the volume corridor provisions of the program as previously delineated in the article. With the application of the revised corridors, it now appears that the FY 1974–5 MAXICAP will be revised upward from 13.85 percent to approximately 14.3 percent.

For FY 1975–76, the parties negotiated an 11.5 percent MAXICAP. Negotiated budgets averaged 10.5 to 11 percent. Although year end data are not yet available, the Blue Cross budget monitoring system indicates that the MAXICAP of 11.5 percent may be slightly exceeded due to volume considerations. However, the end result will be greatly improved over the first year and undoubtedly more favorable than national expectations of hospital cost increases.

FY 1976–77 has just gotten underway. Last spring, the Third Parties and HARI and its sixteen member hospitals agreed to a MAXICAP of 10.5 percent. It appears that budget settlements will be in the magnitude of 10 percent leaving a 0.5 percent reserve to cover possible major contingencies and volume adjustments. The Third Parties are hoping to avoid the problem with volume, and the hospitals will be trying to avoid loss situations. Together the parties are hoping to improve their performance and the program in this third year.

Program Impact

While looking at the potential impact of the program on hospital expenditures in Rhode Island, it must also be realized that the program has gone through a metamorphosis since October 1974 and in reality has been a developmental program. Not only have the volume corridor provisions been revised, but other aspects of the program have changed as well. As problems and conflicts have arisen, the program's participants have met to resolve them by modifying the program so as to meet the demands of the cost containment environment and the needs of the participants. Among other revisions made to the program have been redefinition of the major contingency provision, modification of the patient mix provision, clarification of the use of "gains" under the program, and changes in the appeals process of the program. All of these changes have been made with the intent to keep the program viable and improve upon its operation.

The Prospective Reimbursement program in Rhode Island is a local approach to a national problem of increasing health care needs and demands versus limited health care resources. The emphasis is on containing hospital costs and allocating available health care resources in the most efficient and cost effective manner possible. This is not an easy task for either Blue Cross, the State, or the hospitals themselves. The demands on all parties for improved financial management are great. Responsibilities of the parties have significantly increased with the inception of the program in October 1974. However, it must consistently be noted that the Rhode Island program is a voluntary one. Blue Cross, the State and HARI and its sixteen member hospitals mutually developed the program with a commitment to prove that the voluntary health sector can moderate, if not control, hospital costs without the need for governmental involvement. Experience to date is somewhat limited. Preliminary data do, however, seem to indicate that the program is working to moderate hospital costs and that, given the proper tools and commitment of the parties, the voluntary health sector can, indeed, control itself.

REFERENCES

1. The dollar threshold is based on the size of a hospital's budget.

	Hospital Budget	Annualized Program Dollar Threshold
Group I	$15 million or above	$100,000
II	$10–15 million	$ 75,000
III	$ 5–10 million	$ 50,000
IV	$ 5 million or below	$ 25,000

2. Inpatient Routine Corridor

Patient days up:

Percent Change From Agreed Upon Budget	Marginal or Variable Cost Adjustment to Budgeted Per Diem
0% to 5%	20%
above 5% to 7%	30%
above 7% to 10%	40%
above 10%	Renegotiate expenses and revenues associated with the excess over a 10% change in days.

Patient days down:

Percent Change From Agreed Upon Budget	Marginal or Variable Cost Adjustment to Budgeted Per Diem
0% to 5%	20%
above 5% to 7%	30%
above 7% to 10%	40%
above 10%	Renegotiate expenses and revenues associated with the excess over a 10% change in days

3. Inpatient Ancillary Adjustment

a) If a hospital's actual inpatient ancillary revenue exceeds the budgeted inpatient ancillary revenue, then

FORMULA:

1. $A \times 1.01 = B$
2. $(C - B) \times 0.35 = D$; if $C > B$
3. $[(C - B) \times 0.65] \times E = G$
4. $B + D = F$

KEY:

A = Budgeted Inpatient Ancillary Revenue
B = Adjusted Budgeted Inpatient Ancillary Revenue
C = Actual Inpatient Ancillary Revenue for the Year, Excluding Pre-Admission Testing Related Revenues.
D = Amount that may be added to the expense base for the next fiscal year.
E = Percent of Third Party Purchase Program Days to Total Days.
F = Amount of revenue retention by a hospital.
G = Amount of revenue to be returned to each Third Party.

b) If a hospital's actual inpatient ancillary revenue is less than the budgeted revenue, then

FORMULA: $(A - C) \times 0.65 = D$

KEY:

A = Budgeted Inpatient Ancillary Revenue
C = Actual Inpatient Ancillary Revenue
D = Amount of Revenue over Actual Revenue that a hospital shall receive adjusted for the appropriate RCC

No adjustments will be made to the expense base when actual inpatient revenue is below budget revenue.

4. Outpatient Adjustment

FORMULA: $(C - A) \times 0.60 = D$
$(C - A) \times 0.40 = E$

KEY:

A = Budgeted Outpatient Revenue
C = Actual Outpatient Revenue
D = Amount of Excess Revenue that may be retained; amount that may be added to the Expense Base for the next fiscal year.
E = Amount to be returned to the Third Parties on a pro rata basis based on Program billed charges to total billed charges.

No adjustment will be made to the expense base when actual outpatient revenue is below budget revenue.

OTHER SOURCES

The Prospective Reimbursement Protocol as submitted (and revised) to the Social Security Administration by Blue Cross of Rhode Island, the Hospital Association of Rhode Island, and the Budget Office of the State of Rhode Island, March 25, 1974.

The Rhode Island Prospective Rating Experiment Contract between Blue Cross of Rhode Island and the Budget Office of the State of Rhode Island and the State's sixteen voluntary hospitals. Approved October 7, 1976 by the Blue Cross of Rhode Island Board of Directors.

3

Prospective Rate Setting in Washington State

Frank D. Baker

Topics in this chapter include:

WASHINGTON STATE HOSPITAL COMMISSION

Development

THE WASHINGTON STATE HOSPITAL COMMISSION was established by the State Legislature in 1973. However, events and actions which led to the creation of the Commission as a separate and independent agency of state government dated back a number of years. A brief exploration of the years prior to the creation of the Commission is important in order to understand why the State Legislature, in creating the Commission, ran against the tide of opposition to increased regulatory intervention.

INCREASING COSTS

The pressures ultimately resulting in support for regulatory intervention emanated from three general sources: consumers, payers, and the hospital industry itself. Consumer concerns over the escalation of costs for hospital care were actually focused through the aggregate concerns of organized labor. During the late 1960s and early 1970s, labor representatives became aware that previously negotiated benefits were being eroded by the increasing costs of services in hospitals more rapidly than increased benefit packages could be negotiated. In addition, consumer organizations and citizen's rights activists began expressing alarm at the rate of escalation in hospital charges.

The State Legislature began the impact of increasing costs of hospital care in legislative sessions in the late 1960s. Comparison of appropriation requests to support the State Medical Aid program and the Medicaid programs revealed costs escalating far more rapidly than were the available resources. As a result, the Senate authorized a special interim study during 1969 to address the question of escalating hospital costs and to provide recommendations for the Senate's consideration.

A number of major third party payers also began to express concern regarding escalating hospital charges. Most specifically, federal and state agencies responsible for payments under the Medicare and Medicaid programs, the State Medical Assistance program, and the State Workmen's Compensation Medical Aid program faced increasing critical deficit operations as a result of costs exceeding levels of appropriation.

The hospital industry itself also began to express some concerns in the early 1970s, primarily with regard to input prices and the differential payments imposed by governmental reimbursement programs. The introduction of the federal Economic Stabilization Program in 1971 alleviated at least temporarily the industry's concern regarding input prices, but it also compounded the problems for hospitals resulting from differential payment arrangements. Hospitals found little choice but to attempt to recover these so-called contractual allowances from the private pay patients or from other third party payers.

TECHNOLOGY

These same general interests were also expressing increasing concern over the impact of technological innovation and capacity expansion within the hospital sector. Not only had the decade of the 1960s seen significant increases in the total number of beds within the state, the period had also witnessed a substantial proliferation of technologically innovative capabilities. It was obvious that if the trends continued within another decade the state would have more than twice the capacity necessary to provide appropriate health care services to its population.

These concerns, public and private, consumer and provider, led to legislation introduced in 1971 establishing a statewide health planning program and a state certificate of need program.

Coalition of Interests

It is important to understand this background in order to appreciate the context in which legislation was developed creating the State Hospital Commission. The Hospital Commission was not created in an arbitrary manner, and certainly did not grow out of serious conflicts between hospitals and other interests. To the contrary, the legislation creating the Commission was developed by a coalition of interests representing both the hospitals and patient concerns. The overall intent of the legislation is best described by the introductory section in the legislation itself. This section states:

The primary purpose of this chapter is to promote the economic delivery of high quality and effective hospital health care services to the people by establishing a hospital commission with authority over financial disclosure and budget and prospective rate review and other related matters, which will assure all purchasers of hospital health care services that total hospital costs are reasonably related to total services, that hospital rates are reasonably related to aggregate costs, and that such rates are set equitably among all purchasers of those services without undue discrimination.

The legislation further states that it is essential that an effective cost control program be established which will both enable and motivate hospitals to control their spiralling costs.

Structure

The Commission consists of five members appointed by the Governor and confirmed by the State Senate, and are generally representative of the public as consumers, labor, business, and hospitals. Members serve for four-year terms, and receive no compensation other than reimbursement for their expenses while attending to Commission business.

In addition, an eleven-member technical advisory committee was established by statute, representing the various types of hospitals, the field of accounting and appropriate state government agencies. The Technical Advisory Committee on request of the Commission advises on matters of policy, on rules and regulations proposed by the

The Hospital Commission was not created in an arbitrary manner . . . to the contrary, the legislation creating the Commission was developed by a coalition of interests representing both the hospitals and patient concerns.

Commission, and on analyses and studies of hospital health care costs and related matters. The members of the Technical Advisory Committee also serve without compensation other than reimbursement for expenses incurred in the performance of their duties.

The Commission is supported by eight full-time staff members under the direct supervision of an Executive Director appointed by the Commission. The Commission also has authority to appoint a Deputy Director and a Confidential Secretary, with all other positions filled through the State Personnel system.

Financial Requirements

Prior to implementing its several legislative mandates, the Commission adapted a number of significant policy positions. First, it was concluded that in order to maintain the fiscal viability of hospitals, approved rates should reflect the true financial requirements of each hospital. The financial requirements were identified as including approved operating expenses, deductions from revenues, and an allowance for growth and development when justified.

Operating expenses, in addition to ordinary expenses such as salaries and wages, also were determined to include the net costs related to education programs, patient-related research, depreciation allowance, and interest on long-term indebtedness. The Commission further concluded that contractual allowances resulting from essentially mandated reimbursement programs such as Medicare and Medicaid should also be reflected in approved revenue requirements. Charity and bad debts were treated in the same manner.

While the Commission is mandated by state statute to establish equity of rates and reimbursement, it was clearly recognized that the Commission could not mandate federal reimbursement according to the state system. Obviously, the disallowance of such contractual adjustments would result in rates less than financial needs. The longer range solution clearly is to obtain commitment or authority to mandate that all payers recognize the rates as approved by the Commission. Until accomplished, it is necessary to continue to recognize those enforced contractual allowances.

The Commission also determined that, in addition to the foregoing, financial requirements should consider certain additional potential expenses not otherwise covered. This additional need, termed growth and development, was envisioned as a distinct component unique to each hospital. No minimum level was established but the allowable amount was considered to be a variable totally dependent on the justifiable needs of each hospital. Included in growth and development were such elements as the need for net increases in working capital, acquisition of funds for feasibility studies and planning for shared services, mergers, changes in services, expansion and acquisition of new equipment. Under prescribed circumstances, accumulation of reserves toward balloon payments on debt principal were also considered allowable.

The position regarding growth and development grew out of a desire to develop a close relationship between the health planning process and the rate setting process. Recognizing that an undetermined degree of excess capacity for services exists, the Commission expects the planning process to produce recommendations regarding replacement, expansion and modernization of hospital services which can be directly interpreted through the budget and rate setting decisions of the Commission.

UNIFORM ACCOUNTING SYSTEM

Statutes provide for the establishment of uniform systems of accounting and financial reporting, and for prospective budget and rate review by the Commission. The Commission was instructed by the legislation to first develop and implement the uniform system of accounting for all hospitals in the state, and to allow a phase-in period for that system prior to implementing its authority to prospectively review budgets and rates.

Many articles have been published and many discussions held around the country on the pros and cons of uniform accounting systems for hospitals. Opponents to uniform accounting cite the

Without a uniform set of cost definitions, a prospective regulatory process is severely hampered in its efforts to provide necessary assurances of reasonableness of charges.

need for responsibility accounting unique to each administrative structure of each hospital, and support the alternative of uniform reporting systems. Other points in opposition to uniform accounting systems include the necessity of compliance with a variety of reporting systems mandated by reimbursers, difficulties in relating existing procedures to uniform systems and definitions, problems relating to size, complexity, and capability of various hospitals, and the difficulties of applying uniform systems to both manual and automated accounting processes.

However, without a uniform set of cost definitions, a prospective regulatory process is severely hampered in its efforts to provide necessary assurances of reasonableness of charges. Further, without the basis of uniformity, any comparative analyses can be very misleading, and could result in inequities in budget and rate determination by the regulating agency.

Development

Therefore, the Commission determined that a uniform system of accounting was essential to carry out its legislative mandate, and set out in early 1974 to develop a uniform accounting and reporting system for hospitals. Fortunately, the California Hospital Commission, established in 1971, was concurrently working on the final draft of a proposed uniform accounting system for hospitals. They made their draft material available to the Washington Hospital Commission, and the Commission established a special committee to make recommendations regarding uniform accounting. The committee reviewed the draft material prepared by the California Hospital Commission, various uniform accounting systems proposed in several other states, the American Hospital Association systems, and accounting systems in use by hospitals within the state. After considerable review, the committee selected the California Hospital Commission's system as the basis for the design of a uniform accounting system for Washington hospitals. With careful analysis but minimal modification, a uniform system was recommended by the committee in May 1974.

Drafts of the proposed accounting system were distributed throughout the state, and a series of meetings was conducted by the Commission to explore the proposed new system and to gain additional input from the hospital industry. These conferences, meetings with the Hospital Financial Management Association and the State Hospital Association and other interested groups resulted in further modifications in the proposed system. These modifications were incorporated into a revised draft and ultimately adopted by the Commission effective October 1, 1974, for all hospitals. Each hospital then phased in the new accounting system with its fiscal year beginning on or after October 1, 1974.

Provisions

Provisions of the Washington State Municipal Code define procedures whereby hospital districts can be established by the voters of a defined geographic area, and permit such districts to establish and operate hospitals as public entities. As public agencies under the State Municipal Code, such hospitals are subject to all the fiscal and accounting responsibilities of other municipal corporations within the state. These requirements include compliance with regulations and procedures adopted by the State Auditor regarding proper accounting procedures. The Commission, in developing its uniform accounting system, worked closely with the State Auditor to assure the acceptability of the accounting system. Without agreement between the two state agencies, the thirty-five District Hospitals in Washington would have forced compliance with two different systems. As a result of the joint participation, the State Auditor waived all prior accounting requirements for all district hospitals, and adopted simultaneously, with the Commission, the Uniform Accounting System.

In addition, the Commission worked with the State Hill-Burton agency to assure that the accounting system properly identified charitable services rendered by Hill-Burton assisted hospitals. The accounting system also identifies and defines a separate cost center for medical care evaluation, particularly significant now for identifying costs and revenues relating to PSRO activities.

The accounting system as adopted is based on functional accounting principles, but with sufficient flexibility to adapt to the various responsibility arrangements in any hospital. It is designed not merely as a reporting system, but as a practical accounting system for direct application. It establishes clear and specific definitions of each cost center and revenue center, including defined units of measure. It is adaptable to both automated and manual systems, and will accommodate large and complex hospitals as well as the smaller and less complex institutions.

Consistency

Of greatest significance is the fact that the system is consistent with the AICPA accounting principles and hospital audit guide. Specifically, the system provides for consistent matching of revenues and expenses, including deductions from revenue and revenue recoveries. The system is set up on an accrual basis, and provides for uniform treatment of interdepartmental services. Consistent with the Hospital Guide, AICPA, property, plant and equipment are valued and depreciated at historical costs. Consistent treatment of property, plant and equipment and related liabilities is provided, as well as procedures for dealing with long-term securities and payables.

The system also defines accounting for specific purpose funds, education, research, and financial arrangements between hospitals and hospital-based physicians. The chart of accounts is established on a matched numerical system which by code cross references comparable revenue and expense centers.

UNIFORM BUDGETING AND RATE SETTING SYSTEM

With the adoption and implementation of the uniform accounting system, the Commission's next task was the determination of an appropriate budget input process and a system to identify the appropriateness of requested rates and charges. At the outset, the Commission determined that it was administratively impossible to attempt to regulate every charge in each of the 116 hospitals under the Commission's jurisdiction. To act on a limited set of charges would not meet the statutory responsibilities of assurance of reasonable relationship between services, costs, and rates. After careful consideration and extensive discussions with the Technical Advisory Committee and the Ad Hoc Accounting Advisory Committee, the Commission determined that a uniform budgeting system was essential, not only to meet the requirements of the statutes, but also to assure full and accurate explantion of the total financial requirements of each hospital. Through a request for proposals, the Commission selected an accounting and consulting firm to assist in the development of a uniform budgeting system. The consultant team, together with Commission staff and the Technical Advisory Committee, developed a complete budgeting system for hospitals based on the uniform accounting system.

Policy Questions and Answers

A number of major policy questions faced the Commission in its efforts to translate the accounting information to the rates necessary to assure the financial viability of each hospital. These major policy questions included the definition of total financial requirements, or allowable costs; how to interface with the planning process, especially relating to new services and capital projects; the need to accommodate to both small and large hospitals; the level of detail necessary to meet these expectations; and the overall commitment to the development of a budgeting system to serve as a management tool, rather than simply a document for reporting to the Commission.

Designing the System

With the advice and assistance from the Technical Advisory Committee, the Commission determined as follows:

1. Budgeting is a major management responsibility, and therefore, any budgeting systems designed should have immediate and practical application as a working process.
2. Systems should contain sufficient flexibility to accommodate both large and small hospitals.
3. Budgeting and subsequent rates

should recognize the total financial requirements of each hospital, including deductions from revenue and operating margins.

4. The system should provide for a relationship to the health planning system, specifically through the development of goals and objectives by each hospital in order to relate to the overall plans and goals for the service area.
5. The budgeting system should be a complete budgeting process of cost finding by cost center, identification of financial needs, and a rate setting component to identify appropriate rates based on total financial needs.

Between June and September 1974 these systems were designed, a budgeting manual prepared, forms drafted and instructions completed. Copies of the proposed system, together with an illustration of the systems application, were distributed throughout the state to all hospitals, accounting firms, and other related interests. A series of workshops was held throughout the state to familiarize hospitals with the proposal and to gain their input to the design of the system. These workshops resulted in a number of minor modifications and clarifications. The state HFMA chapter also held several two-day workshops on the budgeting system. In April 1975, the Commission adopted by regulation the revised budgeting system effective with the fiscal years beginning on or after October 1, 1975.

As ultimately designed, the total budgeting and rate setting process includes:

- descriptions of the organization
- operation and contractual arrangements
- statements of goals, objectives and action plans by cost center
- statistical recap of the units of service by cost center
- budgeted direct expenses by cost center
- reclassification expense summary
- a single step-down cost allocation system
- budgeted revenues
- revenue reclassification and,
- revenue and expense summary, the rate setting portion of the overall system.

In addition, the total budgeting system includes a three-year capital expenditure budget, a projected cash flow budget, and projected financial statements. Each budget submittal includes prior year totals, current year information with six months actual and six months estimated, and the budget year projections.

HOSPITAL CLASSIFICATION SYSTEM

Concurrently with the development of the budgeting system, Commission staff undertook the development of a system for classifying, or grouping hospitals. The enabling legislation describes a number of "assurances" which the Commission must provide to the general public. The Commission is charged with assuring the public that hospital costs are related to hospital services and that rates are reasonably related to aggregate costs. The Commission was also instructed to consider the similarities among hospitals, as well as the differences between hospitals in acting on budgets and rate requests. In order to provide these assurances, and to make a reasonable comparison, it was determined by the Commission that cost differences between hospitals should be taken into consideration, and that hospitals should be grouped according to those factors which influence their costs.

Traditional Mechanisms

One mechanism frequently used for establishing groups of hospitals is bed size. Preliminary studies substantiated that a classification system based on bed size alone is not adequate to reflect the similarities and differences among hospitals. While classifying hospitals by bed size has the advantage of simplicity, it cannot recognize such differences as complexity of case mix, mix of physician specialties, differences in areas served, various administrative and organization structures, and resources available within a service area. To recognize the significant variables in addition to bed size which influence hospital cost patterns, the Commission carefully examined the most current research in this area. These included grouping systems proposed by the Social Security Administration[1]; Joseph Phillips[2]; Edwards, Miller and Schumacher[3]; Ralph Berry[4]; and by Shuman, Wolfe, and Hardwick.[5] For various reasons, each of these systems was determined to be inadequate for the Commission's purposes of classification for prospective budget and rate review.

Significant Variables

In addition to a careful review of existing literature and research pertaining to hospital classification, extensive effort was made to obtain information from hospital administrators within Washington State. These discussions repeatedly pointed out to the Commission staff that hospital administrators considered a number of varibles as significant in any classification scheme. Variables most frequently referenced in these discussions were: number of available beds, location, population served, area served, mix of physician specialties on staff, average income of the area served, availability of other staff, control, accreditation, case mix and intensity, access to tax revenues, and age and condition of physical plant.

These variables fall into two categories: exogenous and endogenous. The exogenous variables ("uncontrollable" variables) were considered to be economic, market-related variables which represent constraints on the environment in which the hospital operates and are beyond the immediate control of the hospital. The endogenous variables ("justifiable" variables) focus on factors which influence product mix. A third possible group of performance/outcome variables was excluded from the Washington grouping system. Since one of the purposes of the grouping system is to identify hospitals with unreasonable costs, conceptually performance/outcome variables should not be included, since all the efficient hospitals would tend to be classified in one group and all inefficient hospitals in another.

ENDOGENOUS VARIABLES

These variables focus on the product mix of a hospital, which is a multiproduct firm producing products, or services, in different quantities. The general objective of the grouping system is to classify these hospitals which produce similar products in approximately the same quantity into one group. Therefore, it is necessary to include in the grouping system precise measures which identify hospital output variability. To meet this requirement, the Commission grouping system included a service index as Ralph Berry recommends. But to make the service index more precise, a weighting of services and facilities was developed. The weightings indicate the costlines of the services and facilities in a hospital and were developed by the Downstate New York Reimbursement Evaluation Team.[6] A group of administrators and controllers from the Greater New York Reimbursement Committee were asked to evaluate a list of services according to the costlines of the service. The service index and the weightings include 48 selected services, statistically identified from an original listing of 169 hospital services and service arrangements.

Another important proxy measure for

FIGURE 1. BUDGET REVIEW

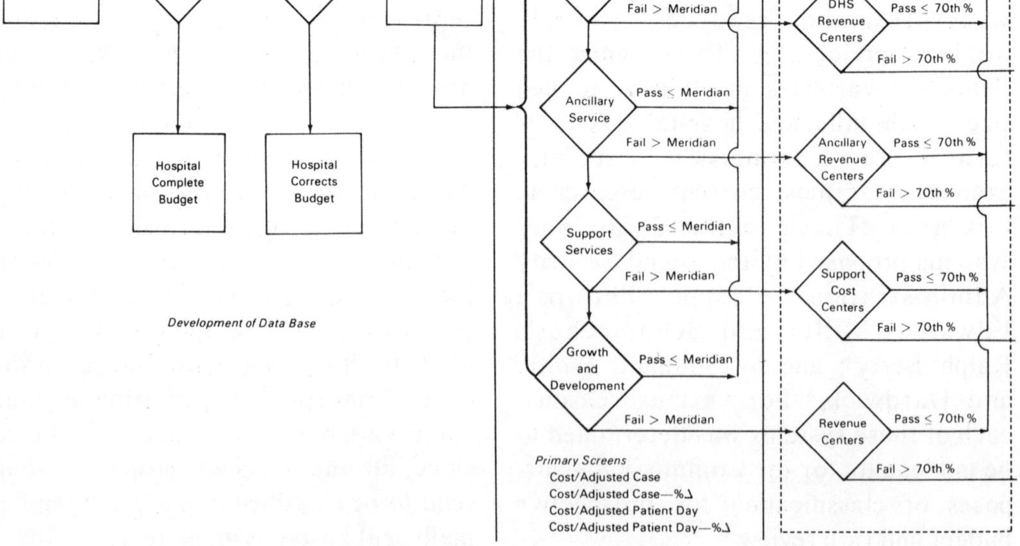

hospital product mix is physician specialty mix. A variety of weightings of physician mix were experimented with and none provided a higher degree of explanation of differentiation than summing the number of physician specialties. Therefore, the latter was used in the grouping system.

Instead of simply indicating the presence or absence of teaching programs, the Washington hospital grouping system established four "teaching" variables: number of interns, number of intern specialities, number of residents, and number of resident specialties. This focus accounts for both the size and the depth of teaching as it relates to product mix.

Medicaid and Medicare patient days as a percent of total patient days were included as a measure of patient and reimbursement variability.

Endogenous Variables (by hospital):

1. Number of available beds
2. Proprietary or nonprofit
3. Government or nongovernment
4. Accredited or not accredited
5. Service Index (based on 48 services)
6. Physician Mix Index—number of specialties
7. Number of interns

SYSTEM: FLOW DIAGRAM

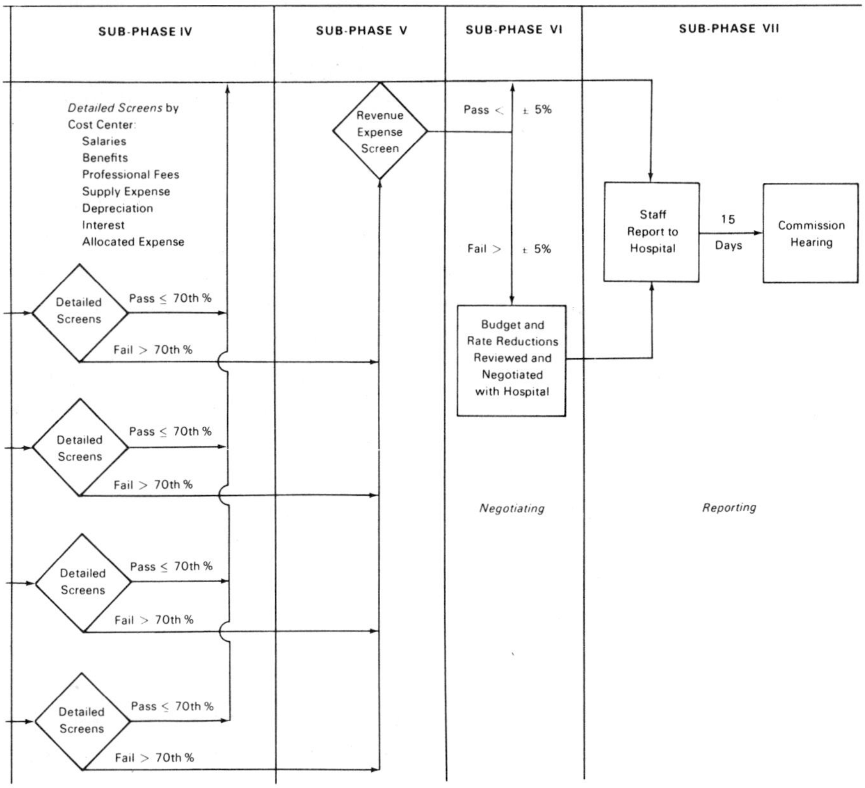

8. Number of intern specialties
9. Number of residents
10. Number of resident specialties
11. Medicare days/total inpatient days
12. Medicaid days/total inpatient days

EXOGENOUS VARIABLES

These economic, market-related variables include factors over which hospitals have no control but which affect their performance. These include primarily socioeconomic and demographic variables which are only meaningful if they reflect the particular characteristics of the region in which the individual hospital is to be found. For this reason, the measurement unit applied to the exogenous variables is the county in which the hospital is located.

Exogenous Variables (by county):

1. Number of physicians per 1000 population
2. Number of hospital beds per 1000 population
3. Percent of population female between 15 and 44
4. Percent population 65 and over
5. Percent urban
6. Median income

The first step in establishing the hospital groupings was to collect the necessary data from hospitals. The hospital responses to a series of specific questions became the data base for the grouping system. No judgments were made in the data as to the accuracy or appropriateness of the information submitted from each hospital. It should be noted that a number of variables such as licensed beds were collected immediately but later eliminated as the system was refined.

Analytical Techniques

A variety of analytical tools were considered and evaluated as to applicability to the problem of hospital classification. The Commission explored the analytical techniques utilized by other investigators dealing with classification of hospitals, and also explored the problem with specialists in operations research. These explorations led to the definite conclusion to test the Cluster Analysis Technique for applicability to hospital classification utilizing the above referenced variables.

It was concluded that cluster analysis is the most appropriate methodology for the following reasons:

a. In this problem, although there are several variables involved, there is not a single "dependent" variable. This is because hospitals are not grouped so as to minimize the variance in one single variable. On the other hand, one needs to group hospitals on the basis of several variables simultaneously. Therefore, all the variables behave like "independent" variables. (These independent variables were further divided into endogenous and exogenous types.) Had there been a single independent variable, then a technique such as Automatic Interaction Detector would be most appropriate for grouping hospitals.

b. The number of ways of classifying items into groups, even for a relatively small number of items, results in an amazingly large number of possibilities. Moreover, the problem is compounded by the fact that usually the number of groups is unknown, so that the total number of possibilities is a sum of Stirling numbers. With such a large number of possible alternatives, the problem of grouping the hospitals appeared to be beyond processing capabilities.

A detailed technical description of the Cluster Analysis rationale and methodology has been prepared by Vandan M. Trivedi, Ph.D., University of Washington, who served as a consultant to the Commission, and is primarily responsible for the analytical methodology for hospital classification.

BUDGET REVIEW AND ANALYSIS

With the completion of the accounting system and the system for classification of hospitals, the next major task facing the Commission and its staff was the design of the actual budget review process. General guidelines for the review of budgets and rates were contained in the original legislation previously described. The Commission had previously determined that its initial focus should be directed to those hospitals exhibiting apparently "high" costs, rather than a detailed line item review of each budget submitted. The Commission was committed to developing realistic analytical procedures without arbitrary standards or preconceived expectations of performance. The Commission was also concerned that the budget review process be realistically achievable within its constraints of seven professional staff and two secretarial support positions. The Commission elected to implement an exceptions review process which would identify potentially high cost operations, and would allow hospitals with apparently lower costs to be approved without a detailed analysis. The Commission was also concerned that the review process include sufficient time for information to be provided back to the hospital prior to the scheduled public hearing on each hospital's budget. Since no historic data base was available due to the adoption of the uniform accounting system, the Commission decided on a budget screening system based on each hospital's budgeted expenses compared to its own peer group.

To avoid the necessity of conducting a detailed review on each budget submitted, it was determined that the screening system should identify those budgets requiring more detailed analysis and those budgets which did not require the additional detailed review. In essence, the screening system was necessary to define "reasonableness" through a series of decision rules which would identify those budgets requiring more intensive analysis. The screening system assists the staff through computerization in focusing on the components of a hospitals budget which appear to be responsible for those cost centers noted as exceptions on the screening. It is also anticipated that this information will aid hospital managers in better understanding their own structure in relation to their peer groups, and also assist the Commission in the review process with hospitals.

The screening system was intended to focus primarily on departmental operating expenses, but the other components of financial requirements were considered equally critical. Net costs related to hospital based education programs were allowed, since at the present time no other sources of funding exist, and such activities were deemed essential by the Commission. Patient-related research activities were similarly viewed, although such expenditures must be demonstrated as directly patient-related and not funded from other sources. As previously referenced, bad debts and contractual adjustments were also considered as allowable expenses. However, both are subjected to a peer group median comparison, analysis of patient mix by payer, and year to year change review. Variance from expected levels require explanation and justification from the hospital.

The Screening System as a Component of Budget Review

The overall goal of a budget screening system must be compatible with the legislative mandate to assure all purchasers that "total hospital costs are reasonably related to total services, that hospital rates are reasonably related to aggregate costs. . . ." The screens therefore focus initially on relating costs to services and follow through to relate costs to the rate requests. The decision rules associated with these screens become an operationalized definition of reasonableness.

Specific objectives of the screening system include:

1. To define "reasonableness" through three types of measures:
   - peer group medians
   - historical trends
   - industry standards
2. To determine, through the reasonableness definition, which hospitals' budgets require further review by the staff and which require no additional review.
3. To maximize the use of data provided by the hospital in the budget package and to reduce as much as possible requests by the Commission for additional data.
4. To obtain the information needed by a staff reviewer to thoroughly evaluate a hospital budget and identify which areas, if any, represent "unreasonable" costs and/or rate requests.
5. To require of hospitals whose budgets fall out of the screens, an explanation of those costs and/or rates which will assist the Commission in the final rate determination.
6. To preserve hospital managerial discretion, consistent with the cost containment objectives of the Commission, by acceptance of those operating budgets that pass the screening process.

The budget screening system is merely one component of the overall budget review process, and is primarily a mechanical process of comparative analysis evaluating each hospital's budget data against comparative data for its own peer group.

The budget screening system is merely one component of the overall budget review process, and is primarily a mechanical process of comparative analysis evaluating each hospital's budget data against comparative data for its own peer group. In order to assure the accuracy and validity of the screening data, the initial phase of the development of a budget data base is a necessary prerequisite to the total review process. Each budget is reviewed by staff for completeness and accuracy prior to input into the data base.

Budgeting and Rate Setting

The budgeting and rate setting process adopted by the Commission provides for a "growth and development" factor as a part of approved expenses and rates. This factor is a variable amount depending on needs and circumstances of each hospital. It is not an automatically approved amount or percentage, but requires documentation and justification. The Commission considers such factors or requirements for funding advanced planning for approved new services or expansion, changes in working capital requirements, and pre-existing commitments. The growth and development allowance provides an additional opportunity to interface planning recommendations with regulatory procedures.

Once the budgets have been reviewed for completeness and accuracy, the data is then used to establish peer group ranges and medians on each of the variables. Each hospital's budget and related data are reviewed against the peer group medians and ranges on each of the selected variables. The complete budget review process can be identified in six sub-phases: data input, preliminary screens, secondary screens, detailed screens, negotiations, and reporting. The screening system has been designed to move along a continuum from very broad aggregate information to more specific and detailed information in an effort to identify the "reasonableness" or "unreasonableness" of projected expenses.

The response and negotiation phase provides each hospital an opportunity to evaluate the results of the screening and their own cost and staffing patterns, and to make adjustments in the budget request prior to the informal hearing before the Commission.

While the screens and their respective decision rules identify and classify hospital costs which appear to be reasonable or unreasonable, it should be pointed out that the response and negotiation phase provides the hospital with an opportunity to explain and justify exceptions noted in the screening process. Noted exceptions may be the result of the inefficiencies and/or excessive costs already known to the hospital, or the exceptions may represent inefficiencies or excessive costs of which the hospital had not been aware prior to the budget review. Exceptions may also represent essential services necessary to maintain the overall services to an area, but which result in costs above peer group medians. The response and negotiation phase provides each hospital an opportunity to evaluate the results of the screening and their own cost and staffing patterns, and to make adjustments in the budget request prior to the informal hearing before the Commission.

Once a hospital's budget has been reviewed at the primary, secondary, or detailed level, it is also subjected to an analysis of the ratio of revenues to expenses. This analysis reviews the relationship between a hospital's requested revenues and its expenses, which includes total operating expenses, deductions from revenue, and growth and development. The analysis is undertaken to satisfy the state legislative mandate that rates be reasonably related to the costs.

If a hospital's budget and rate request is reduced, the rate reductions are negotiated between the hospital and the Commission. Hospital budgets which pass both the cost screens and the revenue to expense ratio screens is subjected to no further review prior to the informal hearing on the hospital's budget. The results of the screening and staff analysis of profile and trend data are provided in a written report to each hospital fifteen days prior to the scheduled informal hearing on its budget request.

Primary Screens

The primary screens focus on operating expenses as defined in the budget package. One aggregate category, total expense, is used and four functional categories (daily hospital services, ancillary services, "other" support services cost centers, growth and development) are reviewed. The first three areas represent an aggregate breakdown of a hospital's total costs into broad functional areas. "Growth and development" expense, unique to the Washington rate setting system and a new concept for some hospitals in the state, is reviewed as a separate cost element.

A total of eighteen expense screens are used in the primary phase. There are four basic measures for all of the categories except growth and development:

1. per adjusted admission as an absolute value,
2. per adjusted admission as a percent change, current year to budget year,
3. per adjusted patient day as an absolute value, and
4. per adjusted patient day as a percent change, current year to budget year.

If a hospital passes the total expense screen and the four functional screens, it then passes to the revenue screen. If it fails total expense it is reviewed in all of the secondary screens. If a hospital passes total expense but fails any of the four functional screens, it is subjected to a secondary review specific to the functional area it has failed.

If a hospital is below or equal to the 50th percentile for its peer group, it passes the screens. For each category, there are four (or two in the case of growth and development) screens. In order to pass the category (e.g., Daily Hospital Services), a hospital must fall below the 51st percentile on all four of the screens.

PRIMARY SCREENS

Total Cost:

1. Total Cost/Adjusted Case Absolute Value
2. Total Cost/Adjusted Case % Change
3. Total Cost/Adjusted Patient Day Absolute Value
4. Total Cost/Adjusted Patient Day % Change

FUNCTIONAL AREAS

Daily Hospital Services:

1. Daily Hospital Services Cost/Case —Absolute Value
2. Daily Hospital Services Cost/Case—% Change
3. DHS Cost/Patient Day—Absolute Value
4. DHS Cost/Patient Day—% Change

Ancillary Services:

1. Ancillary Service/Adjusted Case—Absolute Value
2. Ancillary Service/Adjusted Case—% Change
3. Ancillary Service Cost/Adjusted Patient Day—Absolute Value
4. Ancillary Service Cost/Adjusted Patient Day—% Change

Support Services Cost (administration, plant, dietary, laundry, housekeeping, etc.):

1. Other Costs/Adjusted Case—Absolute Value
2. Other Costs/Adjusted Case—% Change
3. Other Costs/Adjusted Patient Day—Absolute Value
4. Other Costs/Adjusted Patient Day—% Change

Growth and Development:

1. Growth and Development/Adjusted Case—Absolute Value
2. Growth and Development/Adjusted Patient Day—Absolute Value
3. Growth and Development as % of Total Expenses

Secondary Screens

The secondary screens focus on the major cost centers of each aggregate functional area in the case of daily hospital services, ancillary services, and support services. The basic concept behind the secondary screens is to identify which cost centers are causing either a functional category or the aggregate category to fall in the upper half of its peer group. In the case of growth and development, the secondary screens focus on the revenue producing centers reviewed at this level and the specific growth and development factor requested for each revenue center.

The secondary screening is designed to identify projected expenses related to the three major components of hospital costs:

- intensity,
- productivity, and
- input prices.

The following formula generally summarizes the relationship of these components:

Costs/Unit of Output.
= FTEs/Unit of Output × Cost per FTE
+ Non-Salary Costs/Unit of Output.

Therefore, for example, Laboratory Costs per case can be stated as:

Lab Cost/Case = Lab Units of Output/Case × Cost/Unit of Output
(FTEs/Unit of Output × Cost/FTE)

TWO-STEP PROCESS

Secondary screening is actually a two-step process with the second two screens measuring input prices and productivity, and the final two screens measuring intensity and costs. The specific screens by cost center are:

1. Percent change budget year over current year
2. Total expenses/Standard Unit of Measure
3. Number of Standard Units of Measure/Case
4. Total Expenses/FTE
5. Number of Standard Units of Measure/FTE

Two daily hospital service revenue centers are evaluated on the above basic measures: acute care and intensive care. Five ancillary service revenue centers are evaluated: Surgical Services, Central Service, Laboratory, Radiology (includes diagnostic, therapeutic and nuclear medicine or three separate revenue centers) and Pharmacy. Support services cost centers are screened on five cost areas: administration, dietary, housekeeping, laundry and plant. Growth and development is reviewed as a percent of total expense for each of the seven revenue producing cost centers reviewed in the secondary screens. These cost centers were selected on the basis of their significant contribution to total hospital costs.

If a hospital's budget passes the first two secondary screening variables at or below the 70th percentile for its peer group, it is presumed to pass the secondary expense screens. If a cost center fails either of the first two secondary screens, it is further evaluated by the third and fourth variables.

If any cost center is above the 70th percentile on the secondary screening variables for its peer group, it is subjected to a detailed review for that particular cost area. For example, in Acute Care a hospital must be at or below the 70th percentile in all secondary screens to pass. If it is above in any one of the screens, it fails and goes to the detailed screen for Acute Care.

SECONDARY SCREENS

I. DAILY HOSPITAL SERVICES

Intensive Care:

1. Costs/Patient Day, % Change over Current Year
2. Intensive Care Expenses/Patient Day
3. Patient Days/Case (Admission)
4. Intensive Care Expenses/FTE
5. Patient Days/FTE

Acute:

6. Costs/Patient Day, % Change over Current Year
7. Acute Care Expenses/Patient Day
8. Patient Days/Case (Admission)
9. Acute Care Expenses/FTE
10. Patient Days/FTE

II. ANCILLARY

Surgery:

1. Costs/Operating Minute, % Change
2. Surgery Expense/Operating Minute
3. Operating Minutes/Case (Admission)
4. Surgery Expenses/FTE
5. Operating Minutes/FTE

Central Services:

6. Central Service Costs/Patient Day, % Change
7. Central Service Expenses/Patient Day
8. Patient Days/Case
9. Central Service Expenses/FTE
10. Patient Days/FTE

Laboratory:

11. Laboratory Expenses/CAP Units, % Change
12. Laboratory Expenses/CAP Relative Value Unit
13. CAP Relative Value Units/Case
14. Lab Expenses/FTE
15. CAP Relative Value Units/FTE

Radiology:

16. Radiology Expenses/Relative Value Unit, % Change
17. Radiology Expenses/Relative Value Unit
18. Relative Value Units/Case
19. Radiology Expenses/FTE
20. Relative Value Units/FTE

Pharmacy:

21. Pharmacy Expenses/Line Item, % Change
22. Pharmacy Expenses/Line Item
23. Line Items/Case
24. Pharmacy Expenses/FTE
25. Line Items/FTE

III. SUPPORTING SERVICES COST CENTERS

Administration:

1. Administration Expenses/Patient Day, % Change
2. Administration Expenses/Patient Day
3. Administration Expenses/Case
4. Administration Expenses/FTE
5. Patient Days/FTE

Dietary:

6. Dietary Expenses/Meal, % Change
7. Dietary Expenses/Meal
8. Dietary Expenses/Patient Day
9. Dietary Expenses/FTE
10. Patient Days/FTE

Housekeeping:

11. Housekeeping Expenses/Hour, % Change
12. Housekeeping Expenses/Hour
13. Housekeeping Expenses/Foot
14. Housekeeping/FTE
15. Hours of Service/FTE

Laundry:

16. Laundry Expenses/Pound, % Change
17. Laundry Expenses/Pound, Dry and Clean
18. Laundry Expenses/Patient Day
19. Laundry Expenses/FTE
20. Number Pounds/FTE

Plant:

21. Plant Expenses/Square Feet, % Change
22. Plant Expenses/Square Feet
23. Plant Expenses/Case
24. Plant Expenses/FTE
25. Square Feet/FTE

IV. GROWTH AND DEVELOPMENT

1. % of Total Expense of Intensive Care
2. % of Total Expense of Acute Care
3. % of Total Expense of Surgery

4. % of Total Expense of Central Service
5. % of Total Expense of Laboratory
6. % of Total Expense of Radiology
7. % of Total Expense of Pharmacy

Detailed Review

For each cost center, revenue-producing or non-revenue producing, which falls above the 70th percentile in the secondary screens, a detailed review is performed. This review focuses on specific expense categories: salaries, employee benefits, supplies, professional fees, depreciation and interest. It further breaks out the allocated expenses for the particular cost center and evaluates them in relation to the peer group. The purpose of the detailed review is to identify which expenses are causing a hospital cost center to fail the secondary screen.

A variable which is at or below the 70th percentile is considered allowable and will pass. A variable which is above the 70th percentile is considered a failure, and requires further explanation or adjustment by the hospital.

Detailed Review for any or all of the following cost centers:

For any or all of the following cost centers:

Intensive Care, Acute Care, Surgery, Central Services, Laboratory, Radiology, Pharmacy, Administration, Dietary, Housekeeping, Laundry, Plant;

All of the following screens will be used for each cost center:

Salaries: per standard unit, Per FTE, % of Total Expenses

Employee Benefits: Per Standard Unit, Per FTE, as % of Salary Expense

Professional Fees: % of Total Expenses, per Standard Unit of Measure

Supplies Expense: Per Standard Unit

Depreciation Expenses: Per Standard Unit

Interest Expense: Per Standard Unit

Allocated Expenses: Per Standard Unit, % of Total Expenses

Pass-Fail Procedure

If a hospital's budget can pass all eleven detailed screens for an individual cost center, it will be considered a pass and its costs allowed to remain as budgeted. If it fails any one of the costs, the hospital will receive notification by the staff to either provide justification or modify its specific expense to within the 70th percentile. At this point certain negotiations will take place.

Revenue/Expense Screen

In addition to the screening and review of projected expenses, each hospital's budget is also reviewed for the relationship of revenues to expenses by revenue-producing cost centers. This review is to assure that the "rates are reasonably related to aggregate costs," as provided in state statutes. The Commission has accepted in general a relationship of plus or minus 15% as reasonable, but has expressed its intent to progressively narrow this corridor of acceptable relationships. Ultimately, a ratio of revenues to expenses of not more than plus or minus 5% is anticipated. Exceptions to this rule will be subjected to the same subsequent phases as budgets that fail the detailed review of expenses.

Rate Setting

As previously described, the Commission early determined that detailed review and analysis of all prices in all hospitals was impossible. To provide the assurance required in the legislation, the Commission defined "rate" as total financial requirements per revenue center divided by the number of units of service (volume) forecast for that center.

Pricing is a management prerogative, and a hospital responsibility. It is expected that hospital management will set prices to, in aggregate, produce the approved rate setting revenues. In Radiology, for example, the rate might be approved at $2.50 per Relative Value Unit. A procedure equivalent to 10 Relative Value Units would be priced at approximately $25. However, the hospital does have the flexibility to set prices so long as at year-end the hospital meets the Commission's compliance criteria.

Response, Review and Negotiation Phase

The purpose of the response, review and negotiation phase of the budget review is to provide each hospital the opportunity to review the findings and recommendations of Commission staff, to re-analyze its budget and rate requests as submitted, and to either justify the exceptions noted in the budget review or to modify its rate requests prior to the informal hearing on its budget and rate. It is incumbent on each hospital whose budget is noted as having exceptions to utilize the period prior to the informal hearing to thoroughly review the areas identified in the staff findings and recommendations. At this point, hospital management can exercise its management decision prerogatives with regard to which areas can best be adjusted, and which areas can best be justified according to the Commission's review findings.

It is also important that each hospital during this response and negotiation phase further evaluate the relationship of its rate setting revenues to the expenses by revenue center. After the screening and detailed review process is completed, staff findings are prepared and distributed to the hospital and to the Commission. Hospital representatives may provide additional explanatory information to explain or justify a cost noted as an exception, or it may elect to voluntarily reduce its requested expenses.

The reporting phase focuses on providing staff recommendations to the Commission for its approval or modification based upon three information bases: basic financial profile information, the screening process results, and any exceptions formally requested by the hospital.

The basic financial profile includes a ratio analysis of the hospital's financial position comparing it to itself on the basis of current year to budget year, and to industry standards when available. Basic categories of ratios include liquidity, profitability activity and leverage. These are also being used to complete an evaluation of the capital budget request.

FINANCIAL PROFILE

The financial profile includes basic information about the hospital including occupancy, length of stay, percent changes in volume in several revenue centers as well as the aggregate.

Staff findings may also include further review of the budget beyond the variables and the cost centers described in the screening process. For example, an analysis may be made of salary ratios, staffing patterns, changes in staff mix, and other factors in cases where salaries and wages are noted as an exception.

Recommendations are made regarding expenses, ratio of revenues to expenses, deductions from revenues, growth and development, capital expenditures, and rate setting revenues, as well as rates.

PUBLIC HEARING

Each hospital's budget is scheduled for consideration by the Commission at an informal public hearing at which time the staff findings and recommendations and each hospital's response to those findings and recommendations are reviewed by the Commission. Following discussion and exploration of areas of question with representatives of the hospital, the Commission then formally acts on each hospital's budget and rate requests.

After the public hearing, but before the beginning of each hospital's fiscal year, the Commission issues a Decision and Order defining its actions on each hospital's budget and rate request, and identifies its approved operating expenses, deductions from revenue, growth and development, and rate setting revenues. In addition, the Decision and Order defines the rate allowed for each unit of service in each revenue center.

Any hospital that considers the Commission's decision inappropriate may request a formal hearing on its budget and rate request. Such hearings are held before a Hearings Officer, who makes a determination regarding the hospital's request and the Commission's action. If the Commission does not modify its decision after the formal hearing, or if the hospital is still dissatisfied with the final action, it may further appeal the Commission's decision through the state Administration Appeals System to the judiciary process.

Approved Rates and Units of Payment to Hospitals

Once approved by the Commission, the rates per unit of service serve as the basis for pricing services or procedures. While the Commission does not attempt to regulate or monitor each charge by every hospital, hospitals are evaluated at year-end for compliance with the approved rates.

At the present time the approved rates are the unit of payment for all private pay patients, commercially insured, and the State Workmen's Compensation medical program. Medicare and Medicaid continue to reimburse under their cost reimbursement programs, as does Blue Cross.

Year-End Compliance

Within 120 days after the close of its fiscal year, each hospital must file a financial statement, a schedule comparing its actual performance to its budget, and a limited set of supporting schedules. Compliance is determined after allowing for volume variance, and recognizes actual deductions from revenue and the revenues approved for growth and development. Additional revenues are allowed for volumes above forecasts, and reductions are made in revenues for volumes below forecasts. Revenue adjustments due to volume are based on fixed to variable expense ratios determined either by the Commission by peer group, or alternatively from data submitted by a hospital to justify a different fixed or variable ratio. Adjustments are also made to recognize the varying impact of outpatient services on total expenses and revenues. All excess revenue adjustments are applied prospectively to the next fiscal year when a hospital is found to have generated excess revenues.

The entire budget review process from the date of submittal by the hospital to the completion of the public hearing is completed in sixty days or less. While this time frame is extremely tight, experience to date has demonstrated that this can be carried out without sacrifice of quality or opportunity for input and response from the hospital or other interested individuals or organizations.

EXPERIENCE TO DATE

Between May 1974, when the first rough drafts of the uniform accounting system were distributed, to October 1, 1975, a period of only 17 months, hospitals in Washington:

1. Changed to an entirely new chart of accounts and accounting system;
2. Adopted a completely new and extremely complex and detailed budgeting system;
3. Carried out a budgeting and rate setting process, many for the first time;
4. Submitted for the first time a budget and rate request to a new and untested state regulatory agency;
5. Explained and justified their budget and related requests to a public agency, the five-member Commission.

To the credit of every one of the 116 hospitals, they have done an outstanding job of responding to the challenging task. Of greatest importance, the hospitals have participated in every phase of development, have questioned the Commission where indicated, and contributed enormously to the success of the development phase. They have elected to be constructive participants in an effort to improve their system, rather than to challenge progress through legal confrontation.

Certainly there have been, and will continue to be differences between hospitals and the Commission, and this is altogether appropriate. However, these differences focus on specifics; there is no difference in overall goals and objectives.

Between October 1975 and September 1976, the Commission completed the review and took action on 115 budgets and related rates. Original requests for Rate Setting Revenues totalled $650,000,000, including Operating Expenses, Deductions, and Growth and Development. The Commission approved Rate Setting Revenues of $638,000,000, some $12 million less than requested. Approximately one-half of the budgets were approved as submitted, with the balance either voluntarily reduced by the hospital or adjusted by the Commission. To date, none of the 90 hospitals has appealed the Commission's decision.

While prospective payment systems are not viewed as the panacea that will resolve all problems, clearly such systems are a much more effective and equitable alternative to the present disjointed systems of reimbursement.

In addition, many administrators and controllers have commented on the management value of the data derived from the Commission's budget review and analysis. This information, judging from these comments, will become even more valuable to management in future years.

UNRESOLVED PROBLEMS

While the systems now implemented adequately address the expense side of the hospital cost equation, the impact of differential levels of reimbursement remain. Continuation of retrospective cost reimbursement payment systems is counterproductive to the cost containment emphasis of the Commission. Cost reimbursement payment systems provide powerful incentives to hospitals to encourage more units of service to more patients over more days of stay. These payment systems also encourage hospitals to adjust their reporting of costs to maximize reimbursement. While necessary to maintain cash flow and bottom-line position, such actions are hardly consistent with a strong cost management posture.

To meet this problem, the Commission has proposed to the Social Security Administration an experimental prospective reimbursement project. Based on existing systems, the experimental program would establish a prospective payment arrangement, with payment by contract payers determined by an apportionment of each hospital's total budget. If accepted for Medicare, the alternative payment system will also include Medicaid, state Workmen's Compensation, and Blue Cross.

The experience of the State of Washington to date supports the initial position that state regulation of hospital budgets, expenses and rates can be effective and equitable. While the major portion of the developmental phase is completed, many difficult and perplexing problems remain to be resolved. Of greatest significance is that of reimbursement. While prospective payment systems are not viewed as the panacea that will resolve all problems, clearly such systems are a much more effective and equitable alternative to the present disjointed systems of reimbursement.

Regarding regulation in general, the Commission would prefer to see an environment conducive to effective cost containment without regulatory intervention. Given current circumstances and direction of ever increasing governmental payment for hospital services, we are convinced that state-level regulation is the best alternative, and in fact, the key to continued viability of the hospital industry.

REFERENCES

1. The Federal Register, Volume 39, No. 60, March 27, 1974.
2. Phillip, and Ramain, Bureau of Research Services. *A Taxonomy of Community Hospitals* (Chicago: American Hospital Association, June 1974).
3. Edwards, Miller, and Schumacher. "Classification for Community Hospitals by Scope of Services: Four Indexes." *Health Services Research* (Winter 1972).
4. Berry. "On Grouping Hospitals for Economic Analysis." *Inquiry* 10:4 (December 1973).
5. Schuman, Wolfe, and Hardwick. "Predictive Hospital Reimbursement and Evaluation Model." *Inquiry* 9:2.
6. Dowling, Project Director. Unpublished report to the Social Security Administration.
7. Trivedi. *Taxonomy of Short-Term General Hospitals for Control and Equity* (November 1975).

4

Results of Prospective Reimbursement

Clifton R. Gaus

and

Fred J. Hellinger

Topics in this chapter include:

- DEVELOPING PROSPECTIVE RATE REIMBURSEMENT
- EVALUATION METHODS
- EMPIRICAL RESULTS: FOUR STATES
- POLICY CONSIDERATIONS
- THE FUTURE

THERE IS PRESENTLY an intense interest among lawmakers, third party purchasers of health care, and the public in the cost of providing adequate health care. In particular, attention has been focused on the cost of hospitalization. The strategic position of the hospital in our health care system and the predominant role hospital cost increases have played in escalating health care costs as a whole have led to concern over the cost of hospitalization.

In fiscal 1975, the U.S. hospital bill reached nearly $47 billion—three and a half times more than just ten years earlier. While community hospital semi-private room charges have leaped nearly 200 percent in this ten-year span, general prices for consumer goods and services have risen less than 66 percent. Without major changes in hospital financing or delivery, there is no end in sight to the inflation. Mostly as a result of price inflation, Medicare hospital outlays are projected to rise 19.0 percent in 1976 and another 17.4 percent in 1977.

Without major changes in hospital financing or delivery, there is no end in sight to inflation.

DEVELOPING PROSPECTIVE RATE REIMBURSEMENT

In an attempt to control the sky-rocketing cost of hospital care, several states and many Blue Cross plans have implemented prospective rate reimbursement systems. Prospective payment systems set an amount to be paid to hospitals for a unit of hospital services (usually expressed as one day of hospital care) in advance of the period during which care is to be provided. Prospective payment systems replace cost reimbursement, which is still the prevalent method of reimbursement employed by the Medicare and Medicaid programs

Presented to the International Conference on Policies for the Containment of Health Care Costs and Expenditures, The John E. Fogarty International Center, Bethesda, Maryland.

and the majority of Blue Cross plans. Under a cost reimbursement contract, the hospital is automatically and retrospectively paid for all allowable expenses incurred during the fiscal year. Many health care professionals believe that the open-ended nature of cost reimbursement arrangements has provided an incentive for hospitals to expand the volume and complexity of their services without concern for costs or the needs of the public. Advocates of prospective payment systems believe that such reimbursement offers different incentives, as indicated in the following excerpt from the Social Security Amendments of 1972[1]:

> . . . payment determined on a prospective basis offers the promise of encouraging institutional policymakers and managers, through positive financial incentives, as well as the risk of possible loss inherent in that method, to plan, innovate and generally to manage effectively in order to achieve greater financial reward for the provider as well as a lower total cost to programs involved. Prospective reimbursement differs from the present method of reimbursement in that a rate of payment is set in advance of the period over which the rate is to apply. Theoretically, this approach to reimbursement introduces incentives not present under the existing reimbursement method.

Systems in Existence

At the present time, 26 prospective reimbursement systems are in existence in 22 states. These systems are fairly substantial, involving about 25 percent of the nation's hospitals. These systems also take a variety of forms. Eight states have established public rate setting agencies, which approve prospective rates and review requests for modification of those rates. In three of these states special commissions have been specifically organized to perform these functions. In the remaining five, this same power is vested in previously existing public agencies such as health departments. In half these states the rate setting agency is also responsible for purchasing health care services for the public sector.

At the present time, 26 prospective reimbursement systems are in existence in 22 states. These systems are fairly substantial, involving about 25 percent of the nation's hospitals.

In addition to the eight state review systems, 16 of the 74 Blue Cross plans are sponsoring prospective reimbursement systems; and in two states such systems operate along with state programs. In two other states, nonprofit corporations have been established under the sponsorship of state hospital associations to set prospective rates on a voluntary basis.

Support

The Social Security Administration (SSA) was empowered by Congress, through the Social Security Amendments of 1972, to support the development and implementation of prospective reimbursement experiments and to evaluate their effectiveness in containing hospital cost inflation. The Division of

Health Insurance Studies/ORS of the Social Security Administration currently is funding numerous developmental, operational, and evaluative activities in the area of prospective rate setting to determine the desirability of alternative methods of organizing and operating rate setting programs. Presented here is a brief description of the organization and purpose of a few of these projects.

YALE UNIVERSITY

Under contract with SSA, Yale University is now developing a method to describe sets of cases that possess comparable treatment costs based upon diagnosis and surgical procedure. If a rate setting agency based its reimbursement on a per case basis, it would eliminate the incentive to decrease per diem costs (usually accomplished through longer lengths of stay) which exists in reimbursement schemes based on those per diem rates. Such a system will be tested at the Yale–New Haven Hospital after statistically grouping comparable costly cases. The system will also be documented by the contractors to improve its transportability.

RHODE ISLAND

The State of Rhode Island and Rhode Island Blue Cross operate a prospective rate program which, since 1974, has each year set a limit on the total cost of hospital care. This overall limit (MAXICAP is its name in Rhode Island) is arrived at through negotiations between the state of Rhode Island, Rhode Island Blue Cross, and the Hospital Association of Rhode Island. (The MAXICAP was set at 13.85 percent for fiscal year 1975, 11.5 percent for fiscal year 1976, and 10.5 percent for fiscal year 1977.) The Medicare program began paying a portion of the costs of the experiment in 1974 and concomitantly agreed to reimburse hospitals according to prospectively determined rates. These rates are derived from approved hospital budgets, which are reviewed and approved subsequent to the determination of the MAXICAP. Note that the sum of the approved hospital budgets must not exceed the MAXICAP.

UNIVERSITY OF SOUTH CAROLINA

The University of South Carolina presently receives SSA funds to help support a prospective payment experiment employing incentives stemming from management engineering studies to help increase the efficiency within a given hospital department. Hospitals in this experiment are permitted to share in the savings generated through increased efficiency and may use those funds to support new programs that have received planning agency approval. The purpose of this project is to determine whether a hospital can be encouraged through the use of management engineering techniques to implement cost saving programs, if the resulting savings can be used by the hospital to help finance planned new capital expenditures.

BLUE CROSS OF WESTERN PENNSYLVANIA

Blue Cross of Western Pennsylvania operates a combined budget review and formula-based prospective rate program which, in 1974, was expanded to include 16 hospitals. Also in 1974, SSA agreed to cover a portion of the costs of administering and operating the experiment. A brief description of the operation of this budget review-formula system is included in another section of this chapter.

RATE SETTING EXPERIMENTS

Presently, the Division of Health Insurance Studies is in the process of funding several rate setting experiments. A Request for Proposal (RFP) was issued on September 30, 1975, which solicited responses from rate setting agencies and encouraged the respondents to work on either a formula-based or budget review by exception approach. A formula-based approach implies that rates are set automatically on the basis of variables that are exogenous to the individual hospital at the time the rate is set. Consequently, the formula-based approach obviates the necessity of reviewing and analyzing hospital budgets—at least until an appeal is filed. Cost and productivity screens are utilized in the budget review by the exception method of setting rates to identify specific areas in which a hospital possesses unusually high expenditures and, hence, might be inefficient. This method pares down the number of budgets and sections of each budget which must be reviewed by a rate setting agency.

Shortly, contracts will be signed between the Social Security Administration and several rate setting agencies in the hope that these rate setting agencies will develop administratively feasible methods of operating a prospective rate program capable of setting tight, yet equitable, rates. The Division of Health Insurance Studies will issue an RFP for the evaluation of these rate setting agencies to determine whether the experiments have successfully lowered hospital cost inflation without reducing the quality of care.

EVALUATION

Finally, to gather all the information available regarding the impact of prospective payments on hospital costs, the Division of Health Insurance Studies/ORS of the Social Security Administration contracted in 1974 with several research firms to evaluate the effectiveness of seven existing prospective rate systems in six states: Pennsylvania, New York (upstate and downstate), New Jersey, Rhode Island, Indiana, and Michigan. The remainder of this article will present a summary of the results of the evaluations of the prospective payment systems in four states: Pennsylvania, New York, New Jersey, and Rhode Island. The evaluation of the prospective payment system in Michigan, which is being conducted by the University of Michigan's School of Public Health, will be completed in late 1977; the evaluation of the system in Indiana will be submitted this summer.

The following presentation of the findings and implications of the evaluations is divided into three sections: the methods used by evaluators to estimate the cost impact of prospective reimbursement; the specific evaluation results in each of the four states under study; and policy considerations that can be gleaned from the evaluations.

EVALUATION METHODS

Interstate Comparisons

The primary concern of the evaluations was to determine the impact of the prospective payment system on the cost of hospital care. To determine the effectiveness of a prospective payment system, one must know what would have been the behavior of hospitals in the absence of a prospective rate system. Two procedures can be used to isolate and estimate the effect of prospective reimbursement: first, one can compare for a single state the rate of increase of hospital costs before and after the implementation of a prospective rate experiment; and second, one can compare the rate of increase of hospital costs in a state with a prospective rate system (experimental group) with the rate of increase in comparable hospitals in a state lacking a prospective rate system (a control group).

To determine the effectiveness of a prospective payment system, one must know what would have been the behavior of hospitals in the absence of a prospective rate system.

DRAWBACKS

Both these methods have drawbacks. The "before and after" approach does not consider the effects of factors other than the prospective payment system that may have changed during the evaluation period. For example, if a prospective payment system were operational during the same period as the Economic Stabilization Program, it would not be possible to separate the differential impacts of each program through a time-series analysis of data obtained from a single state, even though the data included observations from before and after the implementation of the prospective rate program. In each state under study the prospective rate experiment was operational during the same interval of time as the Economic Stabilization Program (ESP). Consequently, it is necessary to compare hospitals from different states if one is to control for the existence of wage and price controls.

Controlling the Experiment

Interstate comparisons between hospitals, however, implicitly assume that different states possess comparable environments. Since the control groups in these evaluations are used to illustrate what would have occurred in the experimental group in the absence of a prospective rate program, it is important to select control hospitals in a state with similar market characteristics and standards of medical practice. Each evaluator selected a control group of hospitals and employed both an interstate analysis using data from the experimental and control areas and a "before and after" study of data from the experimental state.

COST FUNCTION ANALYSIS

Cost function analysis was used to isolate and estimate the impact of prospective reimbursement in both regressions involving single state time-series data (before and after analysis) and in regressions including data from the prospective reimbursement state and the control state. The use of cost function analysis allowed control for factors other than the reimbursement mechanisms which affect hospital costs (e.g., output levels, case mix intensity, occupancy rate, etc.). Several evaluators accounted for the existence of a prospective reimbursement program through the inclusion among the independent variables of a prospective reimbursement dichotomous variable. The prospective reimbursement variable was set equal to one for hospitals participating in the experiment and to zero for those not in the prospective reimbursement system. An alternative measure of prospective reimbursement employed in the three evaluations was to represent the influence of prospective reimbursement through a variable measuring the proportion of revenue received by a hospital that is subject to the prospective rate. In most experiments the prospective rate was applicable to Blue Cross and Medicaid patients. Medicare continued to reimburse on the basis of costs in all areas, and commercial insurers paid charges usually outside the control of the prospective reimbursement system.

EMPIRICAL RESULTS: FOUR STATES

The presentation of the empirical results of each evaluation will be preceded by a brief description of the organization and scope of the prospective reimbursement programs under evaluation.

Western Pennsylvania

CONTROL OF PER DIEM RATE

Blue Cross of Western Pennsylvania (BCWP) initiated and participated in numerous innovative reimbursement experiments during the past 25 years. Beginning in 1950 BCWP has categorized hospitals in order to set maximum limits for per diem reimbursements, and in July 1971 a prospective payment experiment was implemented. Five hospitals from rural Western Pennsylvania, one of which is a rehabilitation center, volunteered for the experiment. In July 1974 the system was included as an option for all Western Pennsylvania hospitals; eleven hospitals entered the experiment.

The approved per diem rate for each hospital is derived by BCWP from data for the current and the base year. (The base year is two years before the year of the prospective rate and one year before the current year.) Initially, expenses for the base year are divided into operating and nonoperating costs, because the formula restrictions apply solely to operating expenses. Base year operating expenses are divided into three categories: (1) general operations—routine services; (2) general inpatient care—ancillary services; and (3) other expenses—including outpatient services.

To derive the allowable current year operating expenses, the base year general operations expenses per bed, general inpatient care expenses per day, and other expenses are compared with the corresponding values for these categories for the current year. The allowable current year operating expenses are determined using the lower of the hospital's or the composite rate of change for each category. The composite rate of change for this step is the average rate of change for the hospital over the past three years plus the average rate of change for the hospital's group divided by two. (Hospitals are assigned to a group by BCWP according to their location, teaching status, and bed size.)

After determining the allowable current year operating expenses, these expenses are divided into seven natural expense categories (salaries, fees, food, drugs, utilities, maintenance, and other). The budgeted per diem value for each of these categories is compared with an estimate of each category's expense derived by applying the expected inflation rate obtained from Bureau of Labor Statistics (BLS) data. Again, the allowable rate of increase is determined by using the lower of the hospital's or the composite rate of change for each category. The composite rate for this calculation is obtained by adding the budgeted increase for each category and the expected increase due to inflation. This sum is divided by two, which provides the average.

The approved per diem rate is obtained by summing the approved operating per diem rate and the approved nonoperating per diem rate (nonoperating expenses are reviewed and approved by BCWP, but not subject to any maximum formula). In addition, total hospital expenditures are adjusted retroactively. Total reimbursement is limited based on a comparison of the hospital's per diem cost with that of its group. The maximum reimbursable cost per patient day for each hospital is set at a level 12 percent above the group mean cost per patient day.

EVALUATION

The evaluators analyzed data from fiscal years 1971–74 and concluded that the five hospitals which participated in the experiment registered smaller increases in nonphysician-dominated departments (e.g., operation of plant, maintenance, dietary, laundry and linen) than the control hospitals.[2] The ten control hospitals were selected from

The evaluators analyzed data from fiscal years 1971–74 and concluded that the five hospitals which participated in the experiment registered smaller increases in nonphysician-dominated departments than the control hospitals.

Western Pennsylvania on the basis of the population in a county living in a rural area, complexity of services, bed size, percent occupancy, ownership, and the existence of teaching programs. The cost of operating the nonphysician-dominated departments (general service departments) increased 75 percent for the control hospitals and 52 percent for the prospectively reimbursed hospitals during the 1971–74 period. In addition, there was no perceptible difference between the rate of increase in costs for the ancillary departments in the control and the experimental hospitals. The evaluators concluded from this observation that hospital administrators, when faced with the need to control expenditures, were reluctant to implement cuts in ancillary departments, which they felt were important for keeping and attracting physicians.

New Jersey

LIMITED REIMBURSEMENT

New Jersey was among the first of the states to limit reimbursement to hospitals. In 1958, through the authority granted in the 1938 Blue Cross enabling act, the Commissioner of Insurance imposed ceilings on Blue Cross rates of payment. Hospitals were able to appeal for an exception to an Advisory Committee, whose members were appointed by the Commissioner of Insurance. In 1971 the New Jersey legislature passed the Health Care Facilities Act, which aimed at establishing an administrative and regulatory structure to ensure high quality care at reasonable costs. The law resulted in a mandatory prospective rate system, with the gathering, preparation, and analysis of hospital budgets to be performed by staff members of the Hospital Research and Educational Trust (HRET), a subsidiary corporation of the New Jersey Hospital Association. The Advisory Committee to the Commissioner of Insurance was given the responsibility of reviewing, before final approval, per diem rates for Blue Cross and state-supported patients. That committee relied almost entirely on information and analysis provided by the HRET staff concerning the reasonableness of each budget.

The evaluators of the New Jersey prospective rate system concluded that there was no statistically significant relationship between prospective reimbursement and costs, productivity, or quality.

Due partly to the publication of *Bureaucratic Malpractice* (1974), a study by the Center for Analysis of Public Issues attacking the role of HRET in the budget review process, data and analysis for the Advisory Committee are now provided by employees of the state Department of Health. The new system has been in operation since the summer of 1974 and was not analyzed by the evaluator because of the unavailability of data from this period at the time of the evaluation.

EVALUATION

The evaluators of the New Jersey prospective rate system concluded that there was no statistically significant relationship between prospective reimbursement and costs, productivity, or quality.[3] Although the coefficient of the prospective reimbursement variable was insignificant in the estimated cost functions, it was negative. The size of the negative coefficient suggested that the prospective rate program in New Jersey was associated with cost levels two to three percent per year lower for a patient day of care than would have been experienced in the absence of a prospective rate program. These results were robust across a wide variety of linear and log-linear specifications of the cost functions, which included pooled time-series, cross section regressions (hospitals in the Philadelphia area were used as a control group); lagged adjustment models of pooled time-series, cross section regressions, and individual year regressions of the New Jersey and control hospitals.

Rhode Island

BUDGET REVIEW PROCESS

The Director of Business Regulation in Rhode Island regulates Blue Cross rates. In 1970 Rhode Island hospitals presented budgets to the Blue Cross plan which, if implemented, would necessitate a 40 percent increase in insurance rates. Under sustained pressure from the public and the media, the Blue Cross plan asked each member hospital to decrease their proposed expenditures by three percent to an overall rate of 15 percent. The Hospital Association of Rhode Island (HARI) refused to limit planned expenditures and was prepared to help each hospital defend its budget in public hearings. However, after continued bitter attacks from the public and the media, the hospitals agreed to guarantee rates at a level which resulted in a 15 percent increase in revenues. Rhode Island Hospital, the state's largest and most prestigious institution, arrived at a different arrangement with Blue Cross, which included a negotiated budget and a prospective rate for fiscal year 1971.

The budget review process developed by Rhode Island Hospital and the Rhode Island Blue Cross Association for FY 1971 was adopted by the HARI and Blue Cross for implementation for FY 1972 for all Rhode Island hospitals. The program had to be discontinued for FY 1973 because of complications arising from the simultaneous operation of the Economic Stabilization Program (ESP) and the prospective budget review system.

EVALUATION

The control group used in the analysis of prospective reimbursement in Rhode Island was composed of 12 short-term general hospitals in Massachusetts for which case mix data were available from the Professional Activities Studies (PAS) for the time period under investigation (1969–72).[4] The evaluators estimated the impact of prospective reimbursement through the estimation of a cost function with a dummy variable set equal to one for the Rhode Island hospitals in 1971 and 1972. The estimated coefficient for the variable is an estimate of the combined effect of the experiment and the Economic Stabilization Program in the equations using all observations from Rhode Island from 1969–72 and is an estimate for the separate effect of the experiment in using Rhode Island and Massachusetts control group hospitals for 1971 and 1972. The sign of the coefficient for prospective reimbursement was always negative, but only significant in the equations which estimated the combined effect of ESP and prospective reimbursement. For equations measuring only the impact of the experiment, the evaluators found the coefficient of the prospective reimbursement variable to be negative and insignificant. In terms of percentages, the impact of the prospective rate program on inpatient expenditures was estimated to be between two and six percent, depending upon the year and specification of the cost function.

New York

STATISTICAL FORMULA BASE

New York and the state's Blue Cross plans operate the only prospective reimbursement system in the nation which sets prospective rates solely on the basis of statistical formulas; there is no retroactive adjustment. Because of the magnitude of the program and the uniqueness of the experiment, there has been particular interest among health care researchers and policymakers in this program.

The New York prospective rate system began operation in 1970 and does not include a review of hospital budgets or an analysis of their internal operations. It does, however, permit a hospital to file an appeal for the adjustment of its prospective rate after that prospective year. Hospitals complain often and vehemently that severe understaffing of the Division of Health Economics in the state Department of Health has rendered the appeals process hopelessly slow and unpredictable. There are between 150 and 250 hospital appeals submitted each year to the state Department of Health requesting an adjustment of the prospective rate. Often an appeal is pending for a year; in a few instances, the final resolution of an appeal has taken over three years.

SIMILAR PROGRAMS

There are actually three different but similar rate setting programs in New York state that set reimbursement levels. The state Department of Health operates directly the program which establishes hospital rates in New York state for services received by Medicaid recipients, and it delegates to the local Blue Cross plans responsibility for setting Blue Cross payment rates. The Associated Hospital Service (AHS), the downstate Blue Cross plan, sets rates for Blue Cross patients in the 17 lower counties of New York state. The seven upstate Blue Cross plans jointly operate a prospective rate system for their patients in the upstate region.

The state Department of Health, the Associated Hospital Service, and the seven upstate Blue Cross plans' prospective rate systems are remarkably similar in content and process. The prospective rates in the New York systems are derived from actual costs incurred in the base year (two years prior to the prospective year). Routine costs of each hospital in the base year are subject to a ceiling, which is equal to 110 percent of the routine costs for a group of similar hospitals. Any costs in excess of 110 percent of the peer group average are disallowed. The routine costs are then added to ancillary and education costs. Finally, a trend factor, which is derived from a three-year moving average of specified price indices, is applied to arrive at a prospective per diem rate.

Separate evaluations of the impact of the prospective rate program on upstate and downstate New York hospitals were conducted. The findings from the evaluation of the upstate New York hospital study are presented first.

UPSTATE EVALUATION

The major finding of the upstate New York evaluation was that hospital costs grew less rapidly under prospective payment than would have been expected in its absence.[5] However, the estimates on which this finding is based are not statistically significant, suggesting both that there were considerable differences in the responses of the hospitals in upstate New York to the prospective reimbursement formula and that some caution must be exercised in generalizing these results. The estimated coefficients for prospective reimbursement in the cost analysis indicated that total costs per patient day were $.88 lower per year and total costs per case were $11 lower per year due to the prospective reimbursement program. This result, in turn, implies that prospective reimbursement has lowered the average cost per patient day by about one percent per year and the average cost per case by about two percent per year.

DOWNSTATE EVALUATION

The cost containment impact of prospective reimbursement in downstate New York was examined by comparing cost increases in downstate hospitals before and after the introduction of prospective reimbursement with cost increases in a control group comprised of all hospitals in metropolitan Chicago, Cleveland, and Philadelphia.[6] In addition, cost functions were estimated for downstate New York control hospitals that isolated cost trends for two periods, 1968–69 (before prospective reimbursement) and 1969–74 (during prospective reimbursement). It was expected that the cost increase rate in downstate New York under prospective reimbursement would be less than before prospective reimbursement. This expectation was confirmed. However, cost increases also slowed in the control hospitals, presumably due to the Economic Stabilization Program. Therefore, the key question was, did cost increases in downstate New York slow more than in the control hospitals? The evaluators adjusted the cost figures for outpatient visits and the difference in input price increases between regions and found a substantial downward impact on the cost per day and a moderate downward impact on the cost per case attributable to the prospective rate program in downstate New York. The comparison of cost trends showed that after factoring out differences attributable to outpatient visits and input price increases, the average cost per patient day rose 13 percent (2.6 percent per year) for downstate New York hospitals as compared with a rise of 33 percent (6.5 percent per year) for the control hospitals during the 1969–74 period. During this period, the average cost per case in downstate New York increased 10 percent (2.0 percent per year) while the average cost per case in control hospitals rose 21 percent (4.3 percent per year). These findings suggest that prospective reimbursement has lowered the average cost per patient day by about 4 percent per year and lowered the average cost per case by about 2 percent per year. Their findings were supported by the cost function results which indicate that cost per day increases slowed by at least four percent per year and cost per case increases by at least two percent per year as a result of prospective reimbursement. Although the estimates upon which these findings were based were statistically significant, a number of conceptual, data and methodological problems make it prudent to consider these figures only as suggestive.

POLICY CONSIDERATIONS

The evidence from these evaluations suggests that the prospective reimbursement programs under study were moderately successful in lessening the pace of hospital cost inflation. These findings are significant in the sense that

The evidence from these evaluations suggests that the prospective reimbursement programs under study were moderately successful in lessening the pace of hospital cost inflation.

they represent the first careful documentation in the United States that prospective reimbursement has an effect on hospital costs. Although the findings of all five evaluations point in the direction of cost savings, in many cases the results did not pass rigorous statistical tests of significance and, therefore, must be interpreted with caution. Another sobering factor is that, even with highly significant statistics, the magnitude of savings (one to three percent) per year that could be attributed to the systems would not even approach bringing hospital cost increases into line with inflation in other sectors of the economy. In this sense, prospective reimbursement is no panacea, though several percentage points of savings per year compounded over 10 years would be a large factor to taxpayers.

These experiences also indicate that prospective reimbursement is as much a political and legal process as an economic one. The ability and desire of the state's authority to set tight reimbursement rates are contingent on numerous factors, among which are the composition of the body, the nature of the appeals process, the political climate in the state, the nature of participation in the program (voluntary or mandatory), and the rate setting process (budget review, budget review by exception, or formula).

Critical Factors for Effectiveness

Based on these evaluations and other work in prospective reimbursement, one can make certain judgments about factors that are critical to an effective system. First, it is necessary for hospitals in any rate setting system to submit uniform budget and accounting information before, during, and after the prospective rates are established. Second, any system should coordinate health planning and rate setting functions, be it through agreements of the respective organizations or through an integrated organizational model, such as envisioned under the Health Planning Act. A third critical element is to ensure that a prospective payment system focuses not only on per diem cost but on total hospital expenditures, including utilization factors. Evaluation shows that only a slight increase in hospital utilization can offset all the economies from reducing per diem costs. Fourth, it is evident that prospective payment systems will not be fully viable unless they include all payers. This means that, wherever possible, SSA is encouraging and participating in prospective payment systems that include other third party payers such as Medicaid, Blue Cross, and commercial insurers. Fifth, experience has shown that significant cost savings in hospitals will not come about on a purely voluntary basis. Any future system will need to be mandatory to some degree. A number of alternatives are now being considered, short of a complete Federal or state takeover of the rate setting function.

Finally, to make the rate determination process itself less costly, statistical measures must be developed to guide the decision-making process. Individual human judgment by a regulator of detailed hospital budget proposals is cumbersome, costly, and arbitrary. On the other hand, these statistical and economic models of hospital costs are not precise enough to set reimbursement fairly. It would appear that at this time the least costly and most equitable prospective reimbursement system would be a combination of tight statistical formulas and a reasonable exceptions process where judgments about special circumstances could occur.

THE FUTURE

Although it would appear that much is known about hospital cost controls, there is a lot yet to learn. For example, none of the long-range consequences of these systems has been tested; nor have the many other approaches to prospective reimbursement in operation in the United States been evaluated. But, significantly, the focus in this country is on controlling hospital expenditures by controlling per diem costs—a task similar to trying to climb Mt. Everest by hiking from New York City. A prospective reimbursement system that controls hospital costs per case has yet to be implemented and evaluated. Most important, no U.S. reimbursement system has significantly altered the organization of hospital services or retarded the growth of utilization of new services and technology adoption. Since the factors of utilization, service intensity, and technology are major factors in rising hospital expenditures, one must look beyond the reimbursement rate itself for better ways of decreasing utilization and directly limiting supply.

REFERENCES

1. U.S. Senate, Committee on Finance, P.L. 92-603, House Resolution 1, Section 222, 92nd Congress, 1972, p. 62.
2. Applied Management Sciences. *Analysis of Prospective Reimbursement Systems: Western Pennsylvania,* prepared for HEW under Contract HEW-OS-74-226, 1975.
3. Geomet, Inc. *The New Jersey Hospital Prospective Reimbursement Study* (Gaithersburg, Md.: 1974).
4. Thornberry and Zimmerman. *Hospital Cost Control: An Assessment of the Rhode Island Experience with Prospective Reimbursement, 1971 and 1972: Rhode Island Health Services Research,* prepared for HEW under Contract HEW-OS-74-197, 1975.
5. Abt Associates, Inc. *Analysis of Prospective Payment Systems for Upstate New York,* prepared for HEW under Contract HEW-OS-74-261, 1976.
6. University of Washington. *Prospective Reimbursement in Downstate New York and Its Impact on Hospitals* (Seattle, Wash.: 1976).

OTHER SOURCES

1. Bauer. *The Combined Budget Review and Formula Approach to Prospective Reimbursement by the Blue Cross of Western Pennsylvania,* prepared for the Social Security Admin. under grant No. 5-P16-HS00472 from the National Center for Health Services Research and Development (NCHSRD) 1974.
2. Bauer and Clark. *New York: The Formula Approach to Prospective Reimbursement,* prepared for the Social Security Administration under grant No. 5-P16-HS00472 from the NCHSRD 1974. *The Indiana Controlled Charges System.* Prepared for SSA under grant No. 5-P16-HS00472 from the NCHSRD 1974; *The New Jersey Budget Review Program,* prepared for SSA under grant No. 5-P16-HS00472 from the NCHSRD, 1974. And *Budget Review and Prospective Rate Setting for Rhode Island Hospitals,* prepared for the SSA under grant No. 5-P16-HS00472 from the NCHSRD 1974.
3. Center for Analysis of Public Issues. *Bureaucratic Malpractice* (Princeton, N.J.: 1974).
4. Dowling. "Prospective Reimbursement of Hospitals." *Inquiry* 11 (Sept. 1974) p. 168–180.
5. Hellinger. "A Comment on a Proposal for Incentive Reimbursement for Hospitals." *Medical Care* 12 (Feb. 1974).
6. Lave, Lave, and Silverman. "Hospital Cost Functions." *American Economic Review* 60 (June 1970).
7. Lave, Lave, Silverman. "A Proposal for Incentive Reimbursement for Hospitals." *Medical Care* 11 (March–April 1973).
8. Roemer, Moustafa, and Hopkins. "A Proposed Hospital Quality Index: Hospital Death Rate Adjusted for Case Severity." *Health Services Research* (Summer 1968).
9. United States Department of Health, Education and Welfare, Medicare Report No. 92-23 in House Resolution 1, Social Security Amendments 1972.

5

Administrative Responses to Prospective Reimbursement

Robert F. Allison, Ph.D.

Topics in this chapter include:

WITH BOTH major political parties advocating increased federal participation in financing the cost of hospital care, policy makers are investigating alternative methods of controlling hospital costs. Since, historically, changes in hospital costs have corresponded roughly with changes in methods of reimbursement by third parties, attention is currently directed at controlling costs by varying the form of payment. That is, if guaranteeing retroactive payment of full costs itself contributes to increases in costs, will reversing that process by determining in advance what a hospital will receive at the end of its fiscal period moderate cost increases during the period? In such experiments, the interest has been primarily in establishing *whether* costs have been influenced by reimbursement.

As could be expected, administrative officials of hospitals have a different interest and perspective in this matter. While interested in whether prospective reimbursement [PR] influences costs, hospital officials are equally concerned with *how* this occurs. To the skeptical, "hard-headed businessman" official, it is important to know what action hospital administrators took in such experiments to affect costs, if such experiments are to have any value to other hospitals.

This article describes one of the few, if not the only, PR experiment which investigated how hospital officials made cost-influencing changes in response to PR. Although this article relies primarily on the Blue Cross of Michigan experiment, the discussion will not be confined to Michigan, and the emphasis will be on information of value to all hospitals. Given the centrality of the Michigan experiment to the discussion, a brief description of its origin and nature is appropriate.

This research is supported by Contract SSA-PMB-74-344 from the Office of Research and Statistics, Social Security Administration.

DESCRIPTION OF THE MICHIGAN EXPERIMENT

With the passage of Medicare and Medicaid legislation in the mid-1960s and the resulting dramatic increases in hospital costs, interest shifted to control of costs. After a series of Blue Cross rate increases of 16 percent to 19 percent, the state Insurance Commissioner of Michigan in 1970 "strongly encouraged" Blue Cross of Michigan [BCM] to institute PR as a cost control measure. After a delay for the Economic Stabilization Program, BCM began in July 1973 a pilot experiment in eleven community hospitals which had volunteered to be included.

Because some readers might wish to know how these hospitals compare with their own institutions, key descriptive characteristics of the experimental hospitals are presented in Table 5-1.

TABLE 5-1
Experimental Hospital Characteristics
(Averages for all 11 hospitals)
1973

Beds [Range: 34 to 400]	159
Admissions	6254
Length of Stay	7.3
Days covered by Blue Cross	38.3%
Per Diem Cost	$97
Occupancy	81
Scope of Services*	26

*Count of number of services shown in AHA Annual Guide Issues 1973. No university teaching hospitals are in the experiment.

Data Form Package

In the Michigan experiment, each hospital completes a package of data forms and submits them to BCM prior to negotiations. The hospital thus provides detailed reports of its last completed fiscal year, the year to date, estimates of the remainder of the current year, and a budget for the prospective year. BCM reviews these data and meets informally with hospital personnel to resolve nonsubstantive, clerical questions. Although they are chronically behind schedule, formal negotiations are supposed to occur about three months prior to the beginning of the prospective year. In negotiations, several high-level representatives of BCM meet with the administrator, controller, and sometimes other hospital representatives such as the chairman of the board, key officials, and possibly the hospital's external auditor.

Actual negotiations center on the forms completed earlier by the hospital. BCM assumes hospital costs increase primarily because of three factors: inflation, utilization, and productivity. Since BCM feels the hospital can most affect productivity, attention in negotiations is directed at significant changes in departmental administration. When differences of opinion occur, BCM is at a disadvantage to the hospital because of the hospital's "insider" knowledge and the absence of generally accepted productivity standards. Typically, negotiations conclude in a series of offers and counteroffers, separated by caucuses of the negotiating teams. Since this experiment was voluntary, should a hospital have refused to agree to BCM's final offer, the alternative was withdrawal from the experiment. (This never occurred.)

Determining Total Expenses

Throughout the negotiations, total hospital expenses for each hospital are determined in advance. Actual hospital expenses in excess of this contractually fixed amount must be met in full by the hospital. If a hospital is able to keep expenses below that figure, it can retain all savings. Thus, a hospital has both an incentive to avoid losses and a possibility of earning a surplus. The participating hospital receives weekly cash payments from BCM equal to 1/52nd of Blue Cross's share of the total budget. Since all other hospitals receive biweekly checks that vary in amount depending on utilization, this feature of PR contributed greatly in encouraging hospitals to enter the experiment.

Other features of the experiment reduce its potential to provide an incentive to control costs. First, only 38 percent of the average hospital's costs are covered by the contract. Second, many contracts contain provisions for retrospective payment of costs that are unpredictable or uncontrollable, i.e., malpractice insurance premiums or utilization of new services or units. Third, the physicians in these hospitals are neither at risk nor directly involved in this experiment. Since physicians exert primary control over utilization (one of the major determinants of hospital costs), their exclusion diminishes the effectiveness of a PR plan.

Since physicians exert primary control over utilization (one of the major determinants of hospital costs), their exclusion diminishes the effectiveness of a PR plan.

Considering both factors that enhance and factors that diminish the constraining power of this experiment, it seems reasonable to conclude that the Michigan experiment provides only a moderate incentive for hospitals to contain costs. Indeed, this conclusion is consistent with interview responses in which officials in these hospitals indicated that their primary reasons for entering the experiment were not to earn a surplus or to contain costs but to receive the regular weekly checks and to gain expertise in a system they predicted would soon be mandatory for all hospitals. Regardless of the theoretical potential of this PR plan to provide incentive or these respondents' reasons for entering the experiment, the plan has, in practice, motivated officials to behave differently once in the plan. Changes that occurred in these hospitals are examined next.

STRUCTURAL CHANGES

PR and Decision Making

A natural expectation one could hold toward this plan is that it would increase the already high level of "bureaucracy" within hospitals; so, several aspects of hospital operations generally thought to constitute bureaucratization were measured. First, changes in formalization were considered. Formalization is defined as the extent to which standard methods of performance exist, the degree to which they are written, and the extent to which efforts are made to ensure that they are followed in actual practice. Results indicate only an insignificant increase in formalization. Since the increase that did occur was only slightly greater than that of control hospitals, it is clear that PR was not responsible for significant changes in this factor.

It might also be expected that hospitals would employ more personnel specializing in accounting and finance to contend with the added work load associated with PR. Apparently, these hospitals are adding such specialists over time at a rate similar to that occurring in control hospitals. Therefore, one can conclude that thus far PR has not created the need for additional financial specialists.

One might also reason that PR would enhance the power of the central administration over lower level supervisors and *vis à vis* the board and medical staff. Our results to date indicate administrators do not perceive their power in relation to these other groups as having increased. Although they do perceive minor shifts have occurred in their power over individual cost-influencing variables [CIVs], increases have been offset by decreases. Since this is similar to the situation in controls, one can conclude PR has not materially affected the level at which final decisions are made.

Related to the question of the level at which decisions are made is the broader question of the effect of PR on the decision-making structure. Our data indicate the medical staff is the last major decision-making body affected by PR, and the least affected. However, in year two of the experiment physicians were being affected—primarily by being denied new equipment they had failed to include in the budget. One should not conclude, however, that this will reduce costs. The effect is more likely to be the inclusion of such capital purchases in the next budget, not denial of the request. Although the governing boards of these hospitals were virtually unaffected by PR in the first year of the experiment, at least one-half were affected by the end of the second year. Administrators indicated the effects were beneficial (i.e., increasing the board's interest, involvement, and information pertaining to planning, budgeting, and cost control). Clearly this is an "educational effect" of the PR plan.

The first and most affected by PR are the department heads. In year one about 50 percent of the administrators indicated their relations with department heads had been affected. By the end of year two, this figure had increased to over 60 percent. Looking horizontally at the hospital, across functional departments, PR most affects personnel associated with the controller and business office. Looking vertically at the hospital, PR most affects the highest administrative and supervisory levels. Administrators seem to agree that PR is primarily and narrowly a financial program, the success of which depends heavily on the expertise and commitment of department heads.

Education and Improved Practice

In addition to regularized cash flow, the single greatest benefit of this PR plan is its educational effect. The administrative and clerical requirements of participation in any PR plan force improvements in planning, budgeting, and cost control procedures in all but the most well-run hospitals. Such improvements are front-loaded, one-time gains occurring early in the hospital's experience with PR. This is one of the main reasons for the success of PR in Indiana. Being in *any* PR plan over 15 years will improve hospital budgeting practices and cost performance. PR improved existing practices rather than caused hospitals to do entirely new things. Most hospitals have always forecasted, planned, budgeted, and monitored performance. PR, in the study hospitals, caused them to do these things better. Also, poor financial planning was unrelated to hospital size. Respondents were asked what type of hospital could best survive under PR—the anticipated response being large hospitals. They seemed to agree that success within PR is primarily a matter of financial expertise, regardless of hospital size. Observation confirmed their opinions.

The administrative and clerical requirements of participation in any PR plan force improvements in planning, budgeting, and cost control procedures in all but the most well-run hospitals.

Expense and Revenue

It is not too much of an exaggeration to say that under retrospective reimbursement, expenses determine revenues. That is, when all budget requests of the various departments of the hospital are totaled that figure determines what changes will be necessary in the charge structure to generate sufficient revenues to pay expenses. Interviewers asked specifically what they did at that point in budgeting when they found projected expenses exceeded projected revenues: did they reduce budgeted expenses or increase charges? The typical response in both PR hospitals and control hospitals was, as one respondent phrased it, "Put projected expenses and revenues together, then adjust charges accordingly." Only a monopolist can ignore the market in setting budget totals. Our data indicate PR did not materially affect this aspect of budgeting. PR improved utilization and cost estimates, but budget totals were the last, rather than the first, step in budgeting. To paraphrase one respondent, "if the budget components are justified, the budget total will be justified." Of course, in other forms of PR a hospital would begin budgeting knowing the budget total constraining all the components. This is at least one difference between a voluntary PR plan in which budgets are negotiated and other, more rigorous PR plans.

A surprising number of experimental and control hospital officials are, in effect, "cash managers." To them, the real goal is to ensure adequate cash flow rather than recovery of full cost and generation of a surplus. Although it is impossible to document, it seems that a slowdown in Medicaid payment to all Michigan hospitals in recent months had more effect on cost containment than PR. If cash determines costs, restrictions on the timing of payments to hospitals might have as great an impact on hospital costs as restrictions in the size of payments.

Cost Prediction

In hospitals operated by cash managers, the budget is used more for prediction than control. Of course, the avowed purpose of a budget is to constrain actual expenditures. Prospective reimbursement did affect actual expenditures, and the effect seemed to exceed the actual constraint provided by the budget. For example, even though only 37 percent of a hospital's costs might be constrained by the PR contract, officials would act *as if* the entire budget were similarly constrained. Some of this incentive could be due to Medicaid policies unique to Michigan; therefore, these findings should not be overgeneralized. Nevertheless, using budgets to constrain costs, a practice the sophisticated reader simply assumes, is a new experience in some hospitals. One administrator of a control hospital boasted that his actual expenditures were never more than one-half of one percent different from budgeted expenditures; he called his method "variable budgeting." However, "variable" to him meant revising his budget upward each month on the basis of expenditures department heads remembered during the year that they had not reported during the budget preparation! Letting actual costs determine the budget, rather than the reverse, might seem strange to the reader; but it is not so uncommon in hospitals. It seems fair to conclude that PR, perhaps any PR, causes hospital officials to use budgets not only to predict costs but also to control them.

Cost Containment

The data underlying the analysis of the actions taken in PR hospitals to control costs are shown in Table 5-2. Cost-influencing variables (CIVs), a term coined by William L. Dowling,[1] are shown in the first column of the table. These are believed to be among the major determinants of total hospital costs. Each of these CIVs is, in turn, influenced by specific actions of the hospital. For example, to affect efficiency, the hospital might conduct special studies to determine the procedures and type of personnel appropriate for a given task. A lengthy list of actions that affect the 10 CIVs was constructed for this study. For each action the administrator indicated: (a) whether they had already done it ["previous emphasis" column in Table 5-2]; (b) whether they were either just beginning to perform that action or increasing/decreasing their past emphasis on that action; and, (c) how much they thought that particular action affected total hospital costs in the long run ["cost-saving potential"]. The responses for two years of the experiment are averaged and shown in rank order in Table 5-2.

What a hospital is currently doing

TABLE 5-2
Cost-Influencing Actions

CIV	Current Emphasis	Previous Emphasis	Cost-Saving Potential	Administrator's Power
Investments	1	1	10	1
Quality	2	2	3	7
Admissions	3	9	2	6
Scope of Services	4	10	7.5	8
Teaching	5	4	5	4
Length of Stay	6	6	1	5
Case Mix	7	8	9	10
Efficiency	8	5	6	3
Intensity	9	7	4	9
Input Prices	10	3	7.5	2

about cost containment depends on a number of factors, the three most important of which are presented here: previous emphasis, potential for saving costs, and the power to do it. The "administrator's power" refers to the administrator's perception of his/her ability to influence on action *relative* to the medical staff's influence over this action. For example, these administrators felt they had maximum power over the medical staff to control investments in capital and human resources and minimal power to control the types of patients admitted (case mix). The choice of this research design was partly in response to two hypotheses often expressed by academics and practicing managers: some complain that the administrator's failure to take an action that will significantly reduce costs is not due to a lack of will or knowledge but to the fact that the medical staff controls such action; others maintain administrators ignore taking actions that will save money and focus on actions having a low payoff because those are the actions that they have the expertise and power to perform. Available data do not permit a rigorous test of these hypotheses, but perhaps the analysis will provide some fresh insights on the topic.

Examples of actions to control the hospital's investment in human and capital resources are changes in policies regarding plant maintenance, inservice and professional education, etc. Even though these types of actions were emphasized in the past and offered the least potential for cost savings, they are the ones currently being given the most emphasis relative to other actions administrators might take. Administrators also perceive that they had more power to control this CIV than any other. A possible explanation is that administrators are, like the rest of us, creatures of habit and inclined to take the course of least political resistance. These findings might suggest that such expenditures are among the first to be cut or deferred when resources are mildly constrained by PR.

In the broadest sense, it is hard to conceive of an action that does not somehow affect "quality."

Quality Control

In the broadest sense, it is hard to conceive of an action that does not somehow affect "quality." It is also difficult to think of a single action affecting quality that does not simultaneously affect another of the CIVs. As used in this experiment, quality is not a separate CIV but a unit of measure for the other CIVs. Because only physicians may practice medicine, hospitals can only indirectly affect quality—by taking actions affecting the other CIVs. Respondents were asked for their definition of quality, and they defined it primarily in terms of the scope of services offered by the hospital and the type and number of nursing personnel providing bedside nursing care. That is, they see "quality" as a combination of two other CIVs: scope of services and efficiency. The reader should keep these qualifying remarks in mind when interpreting the comments to follow concerning this CIV.

Although actions related to quality received much attention in the past, hospitals continue to give this CIV emphasis. On the surface quality appears to offer the classic example of the CIV having great cost-saving potential, yet being relatively uncontrollable by administration. There are two possible explanations why such actions were stressed despite the fact that administrators perceived the medical staff to have more power than they to control it. First, the types of actions involved are those currently being mandated by government programs and regulations (utilization review). Second, if public statements can be accepted, quality is a central value shared by physicians and administrators; therefore, the administration can act in this area without conflicting with the medical staff.

Other Policy Areas

Compared with other CIVs, admissions received less past emphasis yet offered more potential for saving costs than all but one other CIV. Programs such as outpatient screening and surgery and preadmission certification are examples of actions affecting this CIV. Despite the physician's relative dominance in this policy area, the survey hospitals gave it third highest priority among the ten CIVs. The reason for this seems to be similar to that for quality: government intervention.

Actions related to scope of services have been given the least emphasis in the past, yet they are fourth in current emphasis. This is a policy area in which the cost savings and administrator's power are both perceived to be low. Actions related to this CIV are decisions to add, expand, or contract services or units and to monitor utilization of existing services. A plausible explanation for past inattention to this policy area is the absence of certificate of need legislation. Under PR major changes in services approved by state officials and utilization must be monitored if costs are to be kept within the budget.

Teaching is a CIV in which most of the factors influencing current actions seem fairly consistent. The item includes actions pertaining to both in-service and occupational-type educational programs. It was given moderate emphasis both in the past and currently, has moderate potential for cost savings, and is a policy area where the power of the administration and the medical staff is fairly balanced. In other words, the emphasis on this CIV is about what would be expected.

Length of stay is a CIV offering a good example of the conflict between economic and political determinants of decisions. Despite the fact administrators feel this CIV offers the highest potential for cost savings, only moderate emphasis was and is being given to this policy area. Apparently the lack of emphasis is related to the administrator's perceived inability to take such actions. It is also possible some administrators might not be familiar with policies and programs affecting length of stay (i.e., home care programs, seven-day workweeks, or decreases in turnaround times in lab and x-ray).

The best example of the influence of the dual hierarcy within hospitals is offered by case mix. Administrators feel least able to affect case mix; yet if any CIV is germane to the practice of medicine in hospitals, it is this. Indirectly, hospitals affect case mix through changes in the scope and quality of services offered. More directly, case mix is affected by such actions as policies affecting the composition of the medical staff. It is a CIV that was and is relatively ignored. The administrators

Administrators feel least able to affect case mix; yet if any CIV is germane to the practice of medicine in hospitals, it is this.

surveyed seem to feel relatively powerless to affect this CIV and that the low potential for cost savings is not worth the effort. If administrators were to perceive a large payoff in controlling this policy area, it would clearly invite conflict with the medical staff.

The reader may be surprised to see the low priority given to actions associated with efficiency. This exists despite official perception of this policy area as being highly controllable by administration. Actions typical of those affecting efficiency are merit programs, work studies, use of part-time employees, and admissions scheduling. There has been only moderate emphasis in the past on such actions; they are given even less current emphasis. Apparently the reason for this is the administrator's lack of appreciation for the cost-saving potential in this policy area. Considering the emphasis most college hospital administration programs place on tools to increase efficiency, it is hard to understand the relatively low priority given it by practitioners.

Another explanation for the lack of attention to efficiency is the lack of standards. Hospital officials simply might not recognize that they have efficiency-related problems! As discussed earlier, Blue Cross negotiators gave much emphasis to productivity changes yet were hampered in their efforts by lack of productivity standards. As a bargaining concession, two hospitals in the PR experiment agreed to permit productivity studies by outside consultants paid by Blue Cross. In the absence of such standards, Blue Cross tried in negotiations to disallow budgeted decreases in productivity. In summary, though PR might have stabilized or frozen productivity at historical levels, no data exist to indicate PR improved it. (These conclusions could change as more definitive data are analyzed in the near future.)

"Intensity" refers to the types of diagnostic and therapeutic procedures performed on patients. As the case mix, it is a physician-controlled CIV that was and is given little emphasis. However, unlike case mix, administrators perceive that changes in intensity have relatively more payoff in terms of cost savings. The most logical explanation for this lack of emphasis seems to be the same as that for length of stay, i.e., lack of administrative power *vis à vis* the medical staff.

Actions related to controlling the prices paid for inputs received the least attention of all the CIVs. Since administrators perceive very high control over this policy area, the most obvious explanation is the past high levels of emphasis on this CIV (third out of ten). Either for this reason or from the belief that factors beyond hospital control determine prices and wages, administrators perceived controlling this CIV had a low potential for saving costs.

IMPLICATIONS OF THE MICHIGAN EXPERIMENT

Certain lessons from the Michigan experiment seem obvious. A voluntary PR experiment of the negotiated-budget type is not feasible for two reasons: it is administratively too burdensome on both Blue Cross and hospitals to be feasible on a statewide basis in any but the smallest states, and the voluntary aspect reduces the negotiating leverage of Blue Cross to the point that "negotiations" with hospitals become exercises in cooperative problem-solving. However, one can conclude that procedural requirements of even a voluntary PR plan will improve budgeting practices in all but the most well-run hospitals. Finally, the experiment has increased the cost consciousness and expertise in cost control of Blue Cross officials in Michigan. Given that, historically, Blue Cross officials have been oriented more to serving hospitals than controlling them, this is a major benefit of any PR plan. Beyond these three obvious lessons are three more fundamental lessons from the Michigan experiment.

PR's Incentive Not Enough

First, experience with these hospitals had led one to certain conclusions about the *incentive* value of PR. A major assumption of the Michigan experiment was that the state could control hospital costs through Blue Cross. It appears that such control of only 41 percent of hospital costs provides an inadequate incentive to hospitals. Blue Cross simply cannot do the job alone. To be effective, PR must include Medicare and Medicaid revenues. If this had been done in Michigan, approximately 75 percent of all hospital costs would have been covered by PR. In addition, it is debatable whether any form of cost control is

To be effective, PR must include Medicare and Medicaid revenues. If this had been done in Michigan, approximately 75 percent of all hospital costs would have been covered by PR.

workable since there is much to recommend the view that cost-based reimbursement by Blue Cross, Medicare, and Medicaid is the reason costs are now out of control.

Perceiving CIVs Accurately

Second, it appears cost control depends greatly on the *perception* of factors causing costs. Figure 5-1 presents an understanding of how the major CIVs relate to costs.

Any action taken to control costs is based on some assumption of how that action affects a CIV, which in turn affects costs. Usually these assumptions are implicit rather than explicit. For example, the administrator who devotes most of his time to selection, training, methods improvement, and supervision implicitly assumes efficiency is the major determinant of costs. The administrator who tries to control costs by improving the composition and performance of the medical staff implicitly believes that CIVs related to utilization are the largest determinants of costs (i.e., admissions, case mix, intensity, length of stay). Everyone has such a set of mental assumptions, or a "model."

As shown in Figure 5-1, the length of stay and the types of services received (intensity) are the immediate determinants of cost per case. They require a certain type and quantity of resources

FIGURE 5-1. COST-INFLUENCING VARIABLES

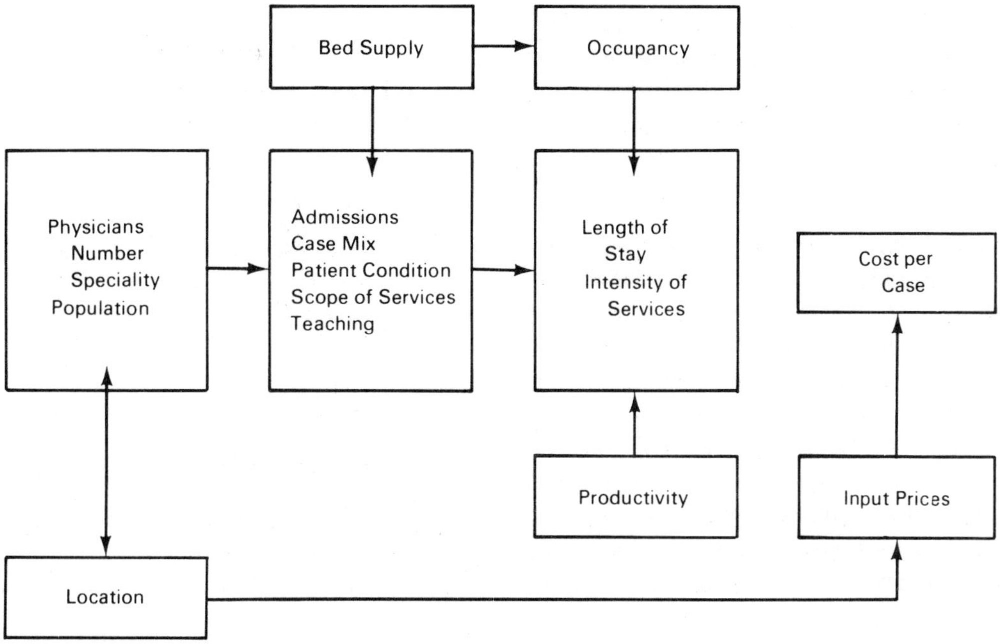

(productivity), which must be purchased at certain unit prices. However, cost per case is not fully controllable by manipulation of only these four CIVs because each is, in turn, influenced by other CIVs. For example, although various "markets" might largely determine input prices, location largely determines the markets relevant to that hospital. The hospital located in midtown Manhattan certainly experiences input price problems different from those of the upstate New York hospital. Similarly, intensity is largely determined by the type of patient admitted (case mix, patient condition). However, the type of patient admitted depends largely on the scope of services available in that hospital and the specialities represented within that hospital's medical staff.

It can be seen that, ultimately, cost per case depends on characteristics of the service area population and the size and specialty composition of the medical staff. The major factors of cost per case are those in the middle row of boxes in the figure, and CIVs to the left are factors influencing those on the right.[2]

Need for Administrator Power

Every administrator realizes the relationship between the medical staff and hospital *revenues.* The current boom in construction of medical office buildings adjacent to hospitals is evidence of this understanding.[3] However, not every administrator sees a comparable relation of the medical staff to *costs.* One rarely meets the administrator who has attempted to control costs by limiting the size or specialty composition of the medical staff. Where actions are taken to control length of stay or case mix, they are usually taken to meet government regulations or to control quality rather than cost. With the exception of the investment CIV, the CIVs currently being emphasized in actions taken by administrators within the PR experiment are roughly consistent with the model shown in Figure 5-1 (see Table 5-2).

It seems clear that administrators now know more about controlling costs than they are able to implement because of a real or perceived lack of *power* to do so. Controlling costs in the short run depends primarily on the variability and controllability of costs. In the short run, variable costs are, by definition, the ones that can be controlled. By these estimates, only 30 percent of all hospital costs are variable in the short run. Also, as has been discussed at length above, certain hospital costs are seen as being

TABLE 5-3
Physician Control of CIVs as Perceived by the Administrator

1. Case Mix	3.65
2. Admissions	3.50
3. Scope of Services	3.45
4. Intensity	3.35
5. Length of Stay	3.25
6. Quality	3.05
7. Teaching	2.65
8. Efficiency	2.30
9. Amenities	2.30
10. Input Prices	2.25
11. Investments in Resources	1.65

Notes: N = 33. Scoring key: 4 = very great influence, 3 = much influence, 2 = some influence, 1 = little influence.

controlled more by the physicians than administration. In Table 5-3 are listed hospital administrators' perceptions of the influence of the medical staff over the CIVs. Scores for administrators of both the experimental and control hospitals for two years of the experiment were combined and averaged in Table 5-1, since the scores were virtually identical for both groups and for both years.

It is clear from Table 5-3 that these administrators have judgmental perception concerning the CIVs that are inherently linked to the practice of medicine. The first five CIVs *are* the major aspects of the practice of medicine in hospitals; and the sixth CIV, quality, is merely another aspect of these five. The last five CIVs are part of the administrative half of the so-called dual hierarchy in hospitals. Given the perceived power of physicians to control certain hospital costs, what part of controllable costs are most controllable by administration? To help answer this question, Table 5-4 was constructed using national averages for short-term, voluntary hospitals in the United States for the interval 1962–66.

TABLE 5-4

Controllability of Expenses: Percent of Total Operating Expenses

Administratively Controlled Departments	**Total**	**Fixed**	**Variable**
Administration and General	.12	.06	.06
Laundry and Linen	.03	.015	.015
Dietary	.09	.045	.045
Housekeeping	.04	.02	.02
Plant Operations	.04	.02	.02
Maintenance	.02	.01	.01
General Nursing	.22	.176	.044
Medical Records	.01	.005	.005
Pharmacy	.04	.02	.02
Education	.01	.005	.005
	.62	.376	.244
Physician-Controlled Departments			
Medical and Surgical Supplies	.05	.04	.01
Operating Room	.04	.032	.008
Delivery Room	.02	.016	.004
Anesthesiology	.02	.016	.004
Radiology	.05	.04	.01
Laboratory	.06	.048	.012
Physical Therapy	.01	.008	.002
Emergency Room	.01	.008	.002
	.27	.216	.054
Subtotals	.89	.592	.298
Depreciation, Interest, Other	.11	.11	
TOTALS	1.00	.702	.298

Although the method, and to some extent the data, in Table 5-4 are partially supported by prior studies, for the most part the analysis is a judgment of the author.[4] It is doubtful that such data have never before been presented despite the importance of this issue to health administration. Administrators probably feel the matter is so obvious it needs no documentation; academics avoid it because of lack of data and the untenable number of assumptions underlying the analysis. Regardless, the basic thrust of the data is unassailable: those with the formal authority to control hospital costs do not have enough power to control them. The estimate in Table 5-4 is that, at most, administrators control less than 25 percent of total hospital costs in the short run. When asked, most administrators and academics will provide much lower estimates.

For PR to be effective, these three conclusions from our research should be given recognition in the plan's design. First, the plan should include Blue Cross, Medicare, and Medicaid revenues to the hospital. Second, the information gap concerning five of the CIVs should be closed. The five CIVs related to quality of medical practice are not now seen primarily as *cost*-influencing variables, but as *quality*-influencing variables. That is, administrative officials are focusing on the five administratively controlled variables having the least impact on costs and letting the medical staff continue to control the five variables having the most impact on costs. Third, for this to occur, administrative officials will need more than education; they will need more power. Certainly an onerous PR plan imposed by the state would increase management's negotiating power with the medical staff; PR *was* well received in these eleven Michigan hospitals, and it brought about the beneficial changes described in this article. It is too soon to know if PR slowed the growth of costs; but it is evident that had the experiment incorporated the three recommended changes, its impact on both actions and costs would have increased considerably.

REFERENCES

1. Dowling, W. L. "Prospective Reimbursement of Hospitals." *Inquiry* 11:3 (September 1974) p. 163–180.
2. Lave, Lave, and Silverman. "A Proposal for Incentive Reimbursement for Hospitals." *Medical Care* 11:2 (March–April 1973) p. 79–90.

   Lave. "The Extent of Role Differentiation Among Hospitals." *Health Services Research* 6:1 (Spring 1971) p. 15–38.

   Shuman, Wolfe, and Hardwick. "Predictive Hospital Reimbursement Evaluation Model." *Inquiry* 9:1 (March 1972) p. 17–33.

   Shuman and Wolfe. "The Use of Case Mix and Case Complexity in Prospective Hospital Reimbursement." [Unpublished manuscript from the University of Pittsburgh] 1974.
3. Toland. "A Hospital Should Own and Operate Its On-Site Medical Office Buildings." *Hospitals* 50:14 (July 16, 1976) p. 80–84.
4. Bauer. *Containing Costs of Health Services Through Incentive Reimbursement* (Boston: Harvard Center for Community Health and Medical Care, Cases in Health Services Series No. 4 December 1973) p. 154–55.

Davis and Foster. *Community Hospitals: Inflation in the Pre-Medicare Period.* (Washington, D.C.: D.H.E.W., Social Security Adm, Office of Research and Statistics, Research Report No. 41, 1972, Table 32. Also: *Six-Month National Comparison for Period Ending December 31, 1973,* Hospital Administrative Services, A.H.A., Chicago, Illinois).

Houser. "Cost Variation With Volume in a Short-Term, Non-Federal General Hospital" [Unpublished Ph.D. dissertation from the University of Wisconsin] 1971.

Davis. "Community Hospital Expenses and Revenues: Pre-Medicare Inflation." D.H.E.W. Pub. No. [SSA] 73-117000, Reprinted from *Social Security Bulletin* (Oct. 1972) p. 10–11.

6

Management Implications of Prospective Rate Setting

John F. Tiscornia

Topics in this chapter include:

OBJECTIVES OF PROSPECTIVE RATE SETTING
HOW DOES PRS FUNCTION?
OPERATIONAL PROBLEMS TO EXPECT UNDER PRS
ALLOCATION OF BAD DEBTS, CHARITY, AND CONTRACTUAL DISCOUNTS
PREPARING TO OPERATE UNDER PRS
DEVELOPMENT OF PRS
PROBLEMS WITH PRS PHILOSOPHY
SOME CONSIDERATIONS

PROSPECTIVE RATE SETTING (PRS) will have a profound and significant impact on the financial viability of hospitals. So administrators and fiscal officers may have a clearer understanding of PRS, the following points will be addressed:

1. *The objectives of prospective rate setting.* What are the advocates of prospective rate setting (PRS) trying to accomplish?
2. *How does PRS function?* A brief review of a case example of PRS in operation and how it affects hospitals.
3. *Operational problems to expect under PRS.* What are the administrative and financial problems hospitals might face under PRS?
4. *Preparing to operate under PRS.* What should the administrator and fiscal officer do to prepare the hospital to operate effectively under PRS?
5. *Development of PRS.* What to strive for when a PRS system is under development.
6. Problems with PRS philosophy. What problems are inherent in the PRS system.
7. *Conclusion.* What to do to maintain hospital financial viability.

The national spotlight is focused on health care costs. They have become the subject of constant and rancorous political debate. Attempts at federal legislation have not solved the problem. Economic Stabilization, which began in the summer of 1971 and ended in the spring of 1974, generally resulted in a decrease in hospital earnings, but not hospital costs.

Traditional Approach and Negative Incentives

The traditional hospital reimbursement approach is a cost reimbursement formula, which pays the cost determined after the dollars are spent. The major deficiencies of this approach are: (1) the more a hospital spends, the more it is paid; (2) the more efficient a hospital becomes, the less it gets paid; (3) payers cannot determine a budget for health costs until after the fiscal year has ended.

To combat these problems negative incentives were imposed. These included limits on routine care cost, paying the lower of cost or charges, and limits on dialysis costs. Many believe the effectiveness of such negative incentives in containing prices is, at best, questionable. Critics still claim that costs have gone up too rapidly and that something must be done to prevent further increases. As a rule, these critics have reviewed only the cost component and have not examined the increase-in-services portion of the equation; but, nevertheless, government agencies and third party payers believe that new price and cost control techniques must be developed to reduce the rate of price increases for health care. In seeking a solution to this problem, federal agencies, state agencies, providers of health insurance, some state hospital associations, and legislators advocate prospective rate setting (PRS).

OBJECTIVES OF PROSPECTIVE RATE SETTING

In the most basic terms, the objective of PRS is to establish an agreed upon rate for all payers, prior to the rendering of service. This is a major conceptual change in paying hospitals. If one were to apply the traditional reimbursement formula to an employee's salary, one could better understand the significance of this change. Under a traditional formula, the employer would ask the employee to report all of his personal expenses at the end of the year, from which he would determine the employee's salary for the year. Under PRS, the employer and employee would agree upon an amount before the year begins. Obviously, under PRS, the employee would have to determine a budget before the year begins and operate within that budget. In the simplest terms, the proponents of PRS advocate that hospitals establish budgets, charge patients based upon budgets, and operate within budgets.

Today, many regulators and health industry personnel believe that PRS will help solve, or at least curtail, the problem of escalating hospital prices. The advocates cite these reasons for changing to PRS:

1. The cost approach used by Medicare and other third parties is not working to control costs.
2. Arbitrary cost ceilings could be eliminated under PRS.
3. Hospitals would be required to live within their rate structures.
4. Payers could better budget for health expenditures since costs and prices would be predetermined.
5. PRS would provide a positive incentive to reduce the rate of price increase for health care services.
6. All payers might be encouraged to

pay the same rate for equal services.

Prompted by the advocates of PRS and the absence of other alternatives, state and federal regulators and other payers are moving rapidly toward some type of PRS. Several states already have PRS, and it is apparent from pending legislation that PRS will be a significant factor for the majority of U.S. hospitals in future years. It is important, however, to understand that PRS is not a universal panacea. There are major problems and pitfalls in the PRS system; therefore, it is imperative that hospital administrators and financial managers understand how PRS functions.

Prompted by the advocates of PRS and the absence of other alternatives, state and federal regulators and other payers are moving rapidly toward some type of PRS.

HOW DOES PRS FUNCTION?

It is relatively easy to discuss the merits of PRS. It is difficult to argue against establishing a budget as a basis for charging patients, and then operating within that budget. However in the conversion from theory to practice, numerous problems do occur. Before discussing these problems and their implications, it may be helpful to provide an example of PRS. This example is taken from one state, and it describes a PRS system from the standpoint of the chief fiscal officer: what it means to him in terms of financial management and his workload. It is not possible to detail the system, but merely to highlight it. Although formats might vary from state to state, the principles remain similar. The following is a brief description of what the fiscal officer must do to comply with a PRS system.

1. *Adopt Uniform Chart of Accounts.* To provide the PRS commission with comparable data, it will be necessary to comply with the chart of accounts defined by the commission. This presents some practical problems: (a) changing of numbers on computer programs, (b) changing of expense distribution numbers, (c) reviewing for conflicts with responsibility accounting, and (d) reviewing for inconsistency in recording data for Medicare.

2. *Adopt Uniform Statistical Procedures.* To provide the PRS commission with comparable data, it will be necessary to define productivity statistics and cost allocation statistics on a uniform basis. To the fiscal officer, this could well mean education of department heads concerning new statistics that must be maintained, and developing several sets of statistics—one for PRS, one for Medicare, and one for management.

3. *Adopt New Budget Forms.* To provide comparability, it is essential that all hospitals use the same forms when submitting budgets to the PRS commission. This could necessitate training department heads in the use of the new forms; developing two sets of budget forms, one for internal budgeting, and the PRS forms for submission to the commission; and separating cost alloca-

tion processes, one for PRS, and one for management.

4. *Preparation for Budgeting.* Prior to preparing the next fiscal year's budget, it is necessary to: (a) insert prior year revenues, expenses, and productivity statistics on the budget forms and complete the cost allocations; (b) insert first six months actual and last six months estimated for current year revenues, expenses, and productivity statistics and complete the cost allocations; and (c) compute the unit cost and unit revenue for each revenue department for each year.

5. *Preparation of Budget.* Now the hospital is ready to complete the PRS forms for the budget year. Once the budget is completed on the PRS forms, a complete cost allocation is performed. It is necessary to compute the unit cost and revenue for each revenue-producing center. The budget, with long and short term goals, must be submitted to the PRS commission 60 days prior to the start of the hospital's fiscal year.

6. *Response to PRS Staff Review.* The PRS staff will review the budget by utilizing some type of screening review process. The hospital will then have a limited time period to respond in writing to the commission staff review, prior to the public hearing.

7. *Public PRS Commission.* At the public hearing the staff comments and the hospital's response will be read. The hospital and the commission staff may provide additional testimony. After the commission votes on acceptance of the budget, the hospital may adjust the rates.

8. *Monitoring Compliance.* During the budget year it will be necessary for the fiscal officer to monitor compliance with the PRS commission-approved plan. This creates an additional responsibility for the accounting personnel.

9. *Uniform Annual Reporting.* After the end of the budget year it will be necessary to prepare a financial report on uniform forms provided by the PRS commission. This report is generally public information and available to whomever requests it. Since the PRS commission needs uniformity of financial data, the hospital cannot merely submit its financial audit report. The fiscal officer must prepare a separate report.

The foregoing is a brief description of a PRS system as seen from the viewpoint of the fiscal officer. The steps outlined are in addition to the normal budget approvals from hospital administration and board of trustees. There is no doubt that a PRS system adds to the workload of the fiscal department. It also requires more sophistication in the preparation and presentation of budgets.

OPERATIONAL PROBLEMS TO EXPECT UNDER PRS

Many problems can surface once a PRS system is initiated. The solution of these problems is vital to the effective administration and financial viability of the hospital.

Management Responsibility Accounting Versus PRS Accounting

The objectives of management accounting and PRS accounting are not necessarily the same. Therefore, hospital administrators must be aware of the conflicts that may arise when PRS is adopted.

PRS—UNIFORM ACCOUNTING AND COMPARABILITY

A PRS system requires uniform accounting and reporting of financial and statistical data to ensure comparability in the budget review and analysis. Peer grouping is merely one method for the PRS commission to compare prospective costs and rates. The data obtained from this peer grouping are utilized to evaluate the costs of the prospective budget. For proper evaluation it is, of course, essential that the peer grouping base data be compiled using uniform methods. Therefore, uniform accounting and reporting are critically important foundations for prospective rate setting. To achieve a high degree of comparability, all discretionary alternatives by hospital management in the recording of financial data and statistics must be eliminated. Even though the most rigorous accounting methods might have been used in gathering the data, it is important that both the PRS commission and hospital administrators realize that such data might not be totally comparable because of the practical limitations of accounting, which is an art rather than a science.

MANAGEMENT RESPONSIBILITY ACCOUNTING

To manage operations properly, hospitals have generally adopted some form of responsibility reporting. Responsibility reporting provides for planning and reporting all costs and revenues to those individuals who are in a position to exercise the most direct control over the costs at each level of responsibility within the organization. Responsibility reporting is designed to follow the individual organization chart of each hospital; so it must have sufficient flexibility to meet the needs of each hospital. Hence, a major issue is the one of uniformity and comparability versus flexibility. Unless all hospitals are organized in the same way, individual hospitals could require and demand a responsibility reporting system that fits its own organization chart. There are many good alternatives in organizing hospitals and reporting the cost of their various departments; but it is important that expenses be budgeted, accumulated, and then reported based upon the organizational chart. Thus, the uniformity requirements of the PRS system make it difficult to utilize this system as a responsibility reporting system for individual hospitals. The conflicts and management problems that can arise are apparent in the following examples taken from a PRS system now in operation.

> *Example 1:* The hospital charges the cost of radiology transporters to the radiology department because they report to the chief technician in that department. The PRS commission requires that these salary costs be charged to routine care.

> *Example 2:* The hospital charges the cost of nurses who administer drugs to pharmacy, because they report to the pharmacist. The PRS commission requires that these salary costs be charged to routine care.

These examples illustrate two possible administrative conflicts and suggest the kinds of questions administrators will have to face. For instance:

1. Should the hospital organizational structure be changed or modified to accommodate the uniformity imposed by the PRS system? This would assume that only one organization chart is best for all hospitals, but this premise is certainly not acceptable to hospital administrators.
2. Should the hospital keep two sets of records; one for the PRS system, and one for hospital administration? Since rates would be set on the PRS system, and costs would be controlled on the hospital administration system, this would necessarily lead to pricing and cost control problems between the hospital, the PRS commission, the public, and other third parties.
3. Should the hospital follow the responsibility reporting system for management and merely reclassify the data for the PRS system? This may require extensive record keeping since both financial and statistical data are required. It will also require a greater degree of financial sophistication on the part of fiscal officers.

Medicare Reimbursement and PRS System

Payment for Medicare patients may or may not become part of the PRS system for hospitals. If it does not, then the fiscal officer must be aware of the effects that changing to a PRS uniform chart of accounts can have on Medicare reimbursement. In 1966, Medicare introduced a set of rules that defined allowable cost and methods of cost allocations. They allowed worksheet adjustments to arrive at defined allowable Medicare costs. The rules and regulations are defined from a Medicare reimbursement standpoint and do not necessarily follow the organization chart and responsibility reporting, nor the PRS system.

This separate regulatory requirement could remain, even with PRS. Thus, the fiscal officer might be required to maintain financial and statistical data that are different from the PRS data and hospital responsibility reporting data. It is apparent that, since the hospital might be required to maintain and report the same financial and statistical data in three separate ways, there must be an increased degree of sophistication in methods of data collection, summarization and reporting.

The adoption of a PRS system uniform chart of accounts could indirectly affect Medicare reimbursement. An actual situation illustrates the problem: A hospital adopted the PRS system chart of accounts on the first day of the fiscal year, and among the many changes for recording revenues and expenses was the following situation. All supply items charged individually to patients in Operating Room were recorded as Central Supply revenue and expense. Previously, this revenue and expense was included in Operating Room. If the hospital merely began recording such detail charges and expenses in Central Supply without keeping separate accounts for these items, it could affect Medicare reimbursement as follows:

1. In the Medicare log, revenue for these items can still be recorded as operating room revenue, yet in the chart of accounts, it is central supply revenue. This inconsistency in matching of revenues could affect Medicare reimbursement.
2. If central supply has a different ratio of charges to cost and a different percentage of Medicare utilization, then Medicare reimbursement might be affected.

When changing to a uniform chart of accounts as required under PRS, hospitals must carefully evaluate the effect of such change on the Medicare reimbursement for each department. Separate accounts must be maintained so reclassifications of revenues and expenses can be made to facilitate preparation of the Medicare cost report on a basis consistent with the prior years. This will require more detailed accounting, but it is essential to evaluate the effect of PRS on Medicare reimbursement. Frequently, fiscal officers do not take the time to provide for this, and in many situations it has adversely affected Medicare reimbursement.

Pricing Policies

One of the primary objectives of PRS is to authorize hospital rates. This will necessarily have a profound impact on traditional hospital pricing policies and practices. In theory, hospitals attempt to set prices based upon the cost of service, but in practice this is difficult to accomplish because of outside influences. Insurance companies, county medical societies, and the news media have carefully scrutinized room rates and publicized increases. Thus, hospitals have found it difficult to accomplish in practice what they, in principle, were advocating. The PRS commission generally requires hospitals to eliminate or reduce cross subsidization and price services based on cost. From a public relations standpoint, this may be difficult for hospital patients to accept.

ELIMINATION OR REDUCTION OF CROSS SUBSIDIZATION

Cross subsidization occurs when a gain from one hospital department is used to offset a loss in another department. The reduction or elimination of cross subsidization has a major impact on pricing policies; it is worth noting what one PRS commission has done and the subsequent impact of its decisions. The law generally states that patients are expected to pay for services based upon the cost of those services. The PRS commission is rapidly eliminating cross subsidization. The commission evaluates whether or not there is cross subsidization by comparing revenues of a particular department with the expenses of the department. These expenses include indirect costs, deductions from revenues, and growth and development. If there is more than a 15 percent cross subsidization, the hospital is asked to review the rates and make adjustments.

This technique will have the effect of reducing the rate of price increase in high profit departments, and increase the rate

Within several years, the elimination of cross subsidization will completely alter the pricing structure for a hospital.

of inflation in departments that are now losing money or breaking even. Within several years this will completely alter the pricing structure for a hospital. The lower the volume in a particular department, the higher the unit cost and price. The PRS commission's action could have the effect of pricing low volume services out of the market. The elimination of cross subsidization, when strictly applied, could have the effect of eliminating services from certain hospitals. The unanswered question is whether the services are needed in that particular hospital. It might be better to let a planning agency determine what services are needed in a particular hospital rather than letting the financial axe cut out certain necessary services. Since cross subsidization is determined after allocating indirect costs to each department and after allocating the deductions from revenue, it is important that hospital financial personnel reevaluate the methods they are using to allocate bad debts, charity, and contractual discounts.

ALLOCATION OF BAD DEBTS, CHARITY, AND CONTRACTUAL DISCOUNTS

It is imperative to a hospital's financial viability that bad debts, charity, and contractual discounts be included in the rate structure. The question then arises as to the allocation of these items to revenue-producing departments. Historically, many hospitals have merely determined the overall percentage of these deductions to gross revenue and allocated it to the departments based upon gross revenues. Under this system, a loss department would be charged with a Medicare discount (whereas a loss department should be credited, since Medicare reimburses on cost). This theory holds as long as the lower of the cost or charges from Medicare is only applied in total. Therefore, to evaluate properly the gain or loss by department, it is apparent that Medicare discounts should be charged on actual basis to those departments that create Medicare discounts. For example, if there is a large profit in the Pharmacy Department, this results in a higher Medicare discount for the hospital. Therefore, Pharmacy should be charged with the actual discounts for Medicare revenue of that department. If routine care is breaking even, then there should be no Medicare discount in that department. The results will be a more realistic accounting method for Medicare discounts and the apparent cross subsidization between departments. This theory would be applicable for all payers who receive discounts because of contractual arrangements. Bad debts and charity should be allocated to the departments on the basis of non-Medicare revenue in each department.

PRS—A Restriction on Administrative Flexibility

The PRS system reduces the flexibility for administrative decision making.

Usually, the PRS commission approves departmental costs, growth and development, and rates. Also, the total hospital expenses, revenues, deductions from revenue, and growth and development are approved. Any upward adjustment of these items generally requires a budget amendment, staff review of the amendment, and a public hearing. This procedure slows the reaction time of administration. It hampers the administration's ability to react quickly to recover from unforeseen circumstances, such as employee strikes.

The administrative procedure for a budget amendment could also reduce the administration's initiative for trying innovative methods to reduce costs during the current year.

Problem of Monitoring Compliance

Under a prospective rate setting system, the monitoring of expenses is vital to the financial survival of the hospital. Weekly, monthly, and quarterly monitoring must be timely and sophisticated enough to determine how well costs conform to prior estimates. If the institution is over budget, and there is no rate recourse, then the administration must take decisive action to reduce the costs. The prospective system puts a greater burden upon the hospital administration to take decisive action and to operate within the budget.

It is usually necessary to provide for some type of year-end compliance test and report. The objective of year-end compliance is to determine the actual variances from the original budget. The budget is necessarily based upon estimates of volume costs. Changes in any one of these will affect the adequacy of the rates originally approved by the PRS commission. If volume exceeds the original estimate, the rates may be too high; or, if volume is lower than estimated, the rates may be too low. Also, effectiveness of management will affect hospital costs. To prevent major rate adjustments at or after year-end, the hospital should closely monitor the effect of these variables. This might present a new set of monitoring criteria to the hospital. The hospital now must apply an external monitoring system, established by the PRS commission, in addition to the in-house management monitoring system.

PREPARING TO OPERATE UNDER PRS

Whether hospitals want it or not, PRS, in one form or another, will soon be a reality for most hospitals. Therefore, administrators and fiscal officers must

Whether hospitals want it or not, PRS, in one form or another, will soon be a reality for most hospitals.

prepare their hospitals for PRS. For adequate preparation, the administration should consider the following:

1. *Discuss PRS With Board of Trustees.* The board must be provided with an understanding of the principles of PRS. They must also understand the short and long range financial implications of PRS. The concepts of PRS must

be compared with the by-laws, goals, and objectives of the hospital, and areas of conflicts isolated for board decision. The board will make final decisions on financial goals and objectives and must be ready to back these decisions with the PRS commission. (This is discussed more below.) To acquaint the hospital board with PRS methods, the following should be considered: in-house training programs, board members attending PRS seminars, board members attending PRS commission meetings, and keeping board members informed of PRS commission activities.

2. *Preparation of Hospital Management.* Financial management on a team basis will be the key to survival under PRS. Therefore, the hospital administrator must prepare the management team for PRS by doing the following:

(a) Conducting in-house training programs on PRS: how the process works, how it affects management, how management decisions affect PRS, and how PRS affects
(b) Sending administrative team personnel to seminars on PRS.
(c) Having administrative team personnel attend PRS meetings.
(d) Training the personnel in the finance department and making sure it is adequately staffed.

3. *Evaluate the Hospital's Budgeting Process.* Since budgeting is the key to financial survival under PRS, it is important that administrators realistically evaluate the strengths and weaknesses of the hospital's current budgeting process. The following questions must be asked, and the answers documented.

(a) Does the hospital have written long and short range goals and a corresponding financial plan?
(b) Are department heads aware of hospital goals?
(c) Do department heads really participate in the budget preparation?
(d) Does the budget responsibility correspond with the organization chart?
(e) Do department heads understand the relationship of budget expenses to rates?
(f) Are timely reports issued, which compare actual results to the budget?
(g) Does the administration take decisive action on a timely basis to correct for variances from budget?
(h) Do administration and department heads understand thoroughly the theory and application of budgeting?
(i) Should in-service training be conducted to teach budgeting theory and application?

These are basic questions, but it is essential that the budget process is securely in place before the hospital encounters the external regulation imposed by PRS. Otherwise, there could be a financial disaster. Once the administrative team is prepared, the next step is the actual budget preparation.

4. *Overall Budget Requirements of PRS.* Hospitals are generally familiar with the normal budget preparation, and thus, all the detail steps of budget preparation will not be repeated. However, PRS could impose additional

budget requirements. The following requirements are taken from an existing PRS system and will generally be included, in one form or another, in most PRS systems:

(a) There must be a definition of the long and short range goals of the hospital and each department.
(b) The hospital should prepare a long and short range plan stating the services and physical facilities needed. This plan should be tied into the appropriate planning agency's plans.
(c) The hospital should prepare a short and long range plan for financing the services and facilities stated in (b). The long range plan should be projected for ten to fifteen years.
(d) The hospital, based upon the short and long range plans, must determine the necessary amount or percentage of growth and development required to accomplish its set goals. This is one area where PRS commissions are tempted to make cuts to achieve a short term decrease in the percentage of rate increase. Therefore, the growth and development requirements must be well documented. The board of trustees and the hospital must be prepared to justify and define, if necessary legally, the amount or percentage of growth and development.

Once these requirements are in place, the budget process under PRS can proceed as described in HOW DOES PRS FUNCTION? However, it is important that the administrator and fiscal officers consider what to do with certain unique aspects of the PRS system and the budget.

5. *Specific and Sometimes Unique Aspects of Budget Requirements.* Certain aspects of the budget that hospital personnel might have previously given only casual review or even ignored will become critically important in budgeting for PRS. Four points are essential: productivity statistics, service units and patient mix, allocating growth and development, and allocating deductions from revenue.

Generally, the PRS commission wants assurance that a hospital is operating efficiently before they approve a rate adjustment. Therefore, it is necessary to budget for productivity based upon the uniform productivity statistics prescribed by the PRS commission.

The hospital administration must educate and train the hospital personnel to budget for expenses based upon productivity statistics. This will force hospital personnel to utilize a flexible budget concept. Total expenses will have to vary, based upon productivity units but with the unit cost remaining relatively constant. All hospital administrators should immediately adopt into the budget process the concept of productivity statistics. Then, when PRS becomes a reality, the hospital personnel will be ready.

The units of service and mix of services are generally different from productivity statistics. For example, a patient day would be a unit of service, but hours per patient day would be the productivity standard. With PRS, the estimate of volume of units of service and the mix of these services becomes extremely critical because the rate is established using these statistics. Thus, hospital administrators must become more proficient in estimating these volumes. This can be accomplished by: (1) reviewing historical patterns and trends, (2) demographic studies, (3) studying the composition of the medical staff, (4) studying the types of services rendered by type of diagnosis, (5) studying the relationship of volume of activity between departments, and (6) monitoring the impact of medical technology upon the demand for hospital services.

The PRS commission will generally require that rates be related to the cost of service by department. Therefore, a method to allocate growth and development to each department must be determined. Should growth and development be allocated on a percentage of expenses by department? If so, what would happen to the growth and development factor in a loss department? Should growth and development be allocated based upon what the traffic will bear? This question is not easily answered, and PRS commissions do not necessarily have a prescribed formula or answer to this imperative question. Thus, hospital administrators must evaluate, make a decision, and document the logic of their approach. Such documentation will be critical in convincing the PRS commission that this question is adequately answered.

The deductions from revenues include bad debts, charity allowances, and contractual discounts. To determine the cost of service properly, these items must be allocated to revenue-producing departments. Hospital administrations typically have not been overly concerned about the method of allocating deductions from revenue, but this allocation becomes critical under PRS. The method discussed above (ALLOCATION OF BAD DEBTS, CHARITY, AND CONTRACTUAL DISCOUNTS) should be utilized.

These are some of the unique aspects that administrators might encounter in preparing a budget for PRS. Now, assume the budget is prepared. What is the next step before submission to the PRS commission?

6. *Isolation and Documentation of Problem Areas.* Once the budget package is ready for submission to the PRS commission, the next step should be a detailed review to isolate those problem areas that may be exposed through the commission review process. This can be accomplished by comparing the budget data with the prior year's peer-grouping information. The administration should, where practical, revise the budget to eliminate such exceptions. This may mean additional discussions with department heads. If budget revisions are not practical, the administration should document the reasons for the exception. Such documentation will be helpful when responding to the commission's budgetary inquiries. After performing this step, the budgetary data are ready for submission to the commission.

7. *An Aggressive Attitude Is Needed.* From the PRS commission's review of the budget, the hospital will receive specific commission decisions about costs and rates. The hospital administration must evaluate the decisions by considering several criteria:

(a) Is a budget revision of costs and rates necessary for certain departments? If so, a revision should be made immediately.

(b) Are the commission's decisions consistent with the overall goals and objectives established by the board of trustees? If not, the hospital must take an aggressive position in responding to such decisions. The hospital should consider three actions: (1) a response to the PRS commission, detailing the conflict between their decisions and the goals of the hospital; (2) if this is not successful, the hospital should request a formal appeal hearing (most PRS systems have an appeals process); (3) If step (2) is not successful, the hospital should consider appropriate legal action.

It is critical that the hospital not passively accept the PRS commission decision if it is in conflict with the goals and objectives of the hospital. Otherwise, the financial viability of the hospital will be seriously impaired.

8. *Hospital Administration Must Have A Budget-Monitoring Process.* Under PRS, the hospital must operate within the approved budget since rates cannot be automatically adjusted to recover cost overruns. This necessitates an increased degree of sophistication for most hospitals if they are to monitor the budget adequately. In addition to the normal requirements, the hospital's budget monitoring system generally must include a timely feedback of variances; the ability to separate, by department, monthly revenue and cost variances due to volume and rate; and the ability to isolate and differentiate between fixed and variable costs. If the hospital is to survive financially, it is vital that the hospital administration make timely decisions on budget variances.

It is critical that the hospital not passively accept the PRS commission decision if it is in conflict with the goals and objectives of the hospital. Otherwise, the financial viability of the hospital will be seriously impaired.

DEVELOPMENT OF PRS

The preceding has provided administrators and controllers with recommendations on what to do to prepare their hospitals for PRS. This assumes that PRS, in one form or another, will soon be a reality. However, in most states, there is still the opportunity to influence the type of system to be initiated. To do this, hospital personnel should:

1. Know the problems inherent in existing PRS systems.
2. Establish active committees in state hospital associations and chapters of HFMA.

3. Be sure that the PRS commission is a separate state or federal agency.
4. Actively participate in drafting legislation that will establish PRS.
5. Make sure that legislation includes a clear statement of financial requirements so guidelines are clear about what should be covered by rates.

Since PRS is a major conceptual change, hospitals must not merely react to legislation. They must plan ahead and participate in making the rules that will govern their financial future. This will require hospital administrators and boards to devote qualified personnel to participate in developing PRS. If they do not take the initiative, others might. To participate in shaping the PRS system, it is necessary to review some of the problems that have been experienced with PRS philosophy.

PROBLEMS WITH PRS PHILOSOPHY

It is difficult to argue with the proponents of PRS who advocate that hospitals establish budgets, operate within budgets, and charge patients based upon budgets. On the surface, this philosophy seems simple and straightforward. However, the application of these basic principles becomes remarkably complex, having a significant impact on the long and short range financial viability of hospitals. Therefore, it is important to discuss the major problems of PRS philosophy, and what its impact will be.

Reduction or Elimination of Growth and Development—the Extinction of Hospitals

Growth and development is defined as the excess of revenues over expenses. Historically, growth and development has been the source of funds for equipment replacements and/or additions to physical facilities and for working capital. Due to the rapid increase in medical technology and because of inflation, depreciation alone is not adequate to replace or modernize physical equipment. Also, many hospitals are using depreciation funds to repay debt. Thus, it is apparent that most hospitals need a growth and development factor.

LONG TERM NEED

PRS commissions, in most cases, are unable to visualize the long term need for growth and development in hospitals. They generally do not recognize the tremendous long term capital requirements of the health care system. They continually emphasize that growth and development will be allowed when a certificate of need is obtained. They fail to recognize that a major building program cannot be financed overnight.

PRS commissions, in most cases, are unable to visualize the long term need for growth and development in hospitals. They generally do not recognize the tremendous long term capital requirements of the health care system.

Funds must be built up over long periods of time if the health care industry is to remain solvent. Generally, PRS commissions have reduced budgeted growth and development amounts for hospitals. The long term effect of such a policy will be to seriously hamper the financial viability of hospitals and to affect the quality of care. Thus, the PRS commission, operating in many instances without an apparent long-range comprehensive plan, could slowly strangle hospitals by reducing or eliminating their growth and development allocations. The risk with this approach is that the financial purse strings may strangle or eliminate certain hospitals which, in the long range, are vitally needed by the community. To minimize this risk, the PRS commission should work closely with a planning agency to determine an overall, long-range, areawide plan regarding which hospitals, if any, will be eliminated. This forthright approach to the problem is more appropriate than is the squeezing of financial resources for all hospitals indiscriminately.

The point is that PRS commissions could appear to be reducing the percentage of increase in hospital rates merely by reducing the amount of the growth and development factor. In essence, this is not a reduction, but only a deferral of price increases to future generations. Such an attitude would give the appearance of short term gains but would leave the replacement of facilities to future legislators. It is clear that PRS commissions must allow a growth and development factor for the long range if hospitals are to maintain their financial viability. If this is not done, there will be a serious deterioration of the physical facilities for health care in the United States.

GROWTH AND DEVELOPMENT FACTOR DEFINED

If the PRS commission law states that a growth and development factor may be included in rates, the next question is definition of terms. The following quotations from Washington state law demonstrate the need for a specific definition of terms:

> NEW SECTION, Sec. 16. To properly carry out its authority the commission shall . . .
>
> (2) permit any nonprofit hospital subject to the provisions of this chapter to charge reasonable rates which will permit the hospital to render effective and efficient service in the public interest and on a solvent basis.
>
> (3) Permit any proprietary profit-making hospital subject to the provisions of this chapter to charge reasonable rates which will permit the hospital to render effective and efficient service in the public interest and which includes an allowance for a fair return to stockholders based upon actual investment or the fair value of the investment, whichever is less . . .
>
> (5) Permit, in considering a request for change in or initiating a review of rate schedules or other charges, any hospital subject to the provisions of this chapter to charge rates which will in the aggregate produce sufficient total revenue for the hospital to meet all of the reasonable obligations specified in this chapter.

The definition of such terms as "on a

solvent basis," "allowance for a fair return to stockholders," "to meet all of the reasonable obligations" becomes a crucial problem. The law uses generalized terms that are then negotiated between the PRS commission and hospitals. For example, "on a solvent basis" could mean that an adequate growth and development factor is needed for the long range replacement of the physical facility. Yet most PRS commissions are not willing to recognize the long range need for growth and development.

In helping to shape PRS system laws, hospitals must evaluate the desirability of having the specific definition of such terms included in the law itself. It might take longer to develop the law or the PRS system, but the foundation will be built on solid ground. Also, if terms are not defined in the law itself, it could be necessary to define such terms later in court, requiring expensive and time-consuming litigation.

Capital Requirements and Depreciation

PRS commissions and the advocates of PRS sometimes confuse capital requirements with depreciation. Thus, it is important to distinguish between these two terms. Depreciation is the allocation of tangible assets over their estimated useful lifetime. In essence, depreciation is the using up of a tangible asset. Capital represents the investment in the hospital by the community, patients, government, and various other sources. Debt is not capital since it must be repaid.

It is important for PRS commissions to realize that a responsibility which most boards of trustees take quite seriously is that of preserving the capital funds entrusted to them. They believe that the hospital's capital is a basic requirement for service to the community; and, unless such capital is preserved, there is no great likelihood that the service can be preserved. Most trustees believe that donors of capital funds imply, by the nature of their gift, that the trustees will preserve the equity. In the event a hospital were not needed, the trustees would presumably use the capital to build a needed hospital elsewhere or would turn the funds over to an organization which could use them to discharge the trustees' responsibility to the community and to the original donors of the funds. Therefore, trustees must preserve the capital funds entrusted to their care. If the PRS commission directly or indirectly usurps the responsibilities of trustees, this would constitute a confiscation of capital by a regulatory agency. Hospitals must prevent such a situation, or the result will be the financial downfall of the health care system.

It is important for PRS commissions to realize that a responsibility which most boards of trustees take quite seriously is that of preserving the capital funds entrusted to them.

Hospital Financing

Sources of hospital financing include growth and development, grants, contributions, and loans. However, loans must be repaid and, thus, cannot be considered a permanent source. The use of debt to finance hospital construction has become more prevalent in recent years. It is important that hospitals explain to lenders the PRS system and the implications it has on debt repayment. Otherwise, they may view it as adding to the risk of a loan and seek other places for their money. If the PRS system is not structured properly, the lenders' concern, in fact, may be valid. This could create a shortage of funds and drastically increase interest rates for hospitals.

Rate Setting Equitably Among All Purchasers

One objective of most PRS systems is to set rates equitably among all purchasers of services. This can be seen in the following quote taken from the Washington State law:

> NEW SECTION, Sec. 2. The primary purpose of this chapter is to promote the economic delivery of high quality and effective hospital health care services to the people by establishing a hospital commission with authority over financial disclosure and budget and prospective rate review and other related matters, which will assure all purchasers of hospital health care services that total hospital costs are reasonably related to aggregate costs, and that such rates are set equitably among all purchasers of these services without undue discrimination.

A literal interpretation means that all third party payers should pay the same rate the private patient is expected to pay. Thus, prior to the initiation of a PRS system, the commission should obtain such agreement from all third party payers. In several cases, this was not done until after the program was in existence for a year or more. This does not meet the purpose as defined above; hospitals should attempt, through close cooperation with third party payers and the PRS commission, to obtain agreements before the PRS system is initiated.

Overregulation

A major consideration of any PRS system is overregulation. If the PRS commission reduces or eliminates administrative prerogatives, initiative will be stifled; creativity will cease. Hospitals must guard against any PRS system that substitutes a commission's regulations for an administration's responsibility to act wisely. Adequate safeguards must be written into the laws.

The Board of Trustees' Loss of Authority

A major problem is that the PRS commission might reduce the authority of the board of trustees yet leave the board with full responsibility for the institution. A few examples will demonstrate this point.

(a) One PRS commission decided that the hospital should borrow $200,000 for a project, rather than earn the money in the budget year, as decided by the board of trustees.

(b) The PRS commission could decide that nonoperating revenues, including contributions, be offset against rates. This could be contrary to the board policies.

(c) The PRS commission might not allow sufficient growth and development funds to preserve the capital of the hospital. Thus, trustees will not be able to fulfill their responsibility of preserving the purchasing power of the dollars of capital entrusted to them.

(d) The PRS commission might force hospitals to close, merge, or consolidate services even though this conflicts with the goals and objectives of the hospital.

These are but a few examples that substitute the judgment of the commission for that of individual hospital trustees and administration. If such incidents happen frequently, it will do much to discourage the trustees' interest in their hospitals. This, of course, could mean the reduction or elimination of community support.

SOME CONSIDERATIONS

The critics of the current health care system claim that industrywide changes are necessary to curb the increases in hospital costs and rates. PRS will inevitably be a major factor in such change. However, the financial implications and administrative problems of PRS, as discussed in this article, must be considered if PRS is to be successful. In the meantime, hospitals must prepare for PRS by doing the following:

1. Participating actively in the development of any legislation establishing PRS.
2. Preparing the board of trustees and hospital administrators for managing under the PRS system.
3. Developing long and short range financial plans.
4. Improving the budgetary, reporting, and financial management process.
5. Reviewing the productivity statistics to ensure an efficient operation.
6. Establishing a policy for financial viability and utilizing an aggressive attitude to maintain it. This should include the goals and objectives for growth and development funds and, thus, maintenance of capital.

The above steps are vital for the financial survival of hospitals under PRS.

7

Information Needs for Hospital Rate Setting

Katharine G. Bauer

Topics in this chapter include:

GREAT EXPECTATIONS

THE BELIEF is widely shared that external reviewers or regulatory bodies will be able to establish rates in a manner that will put the brakes on hospital cost increases while still ensuring that the public has access to good quality hospital care. Further, along with the planning and utilization review controls already specified in P.L. 92-603 and P.L. 93-641, rate setting is seen as an instrument for arresting the seemingly inexorable rise of health care services as a percentage of the nation's gross national product—from 5.2 percent in 1969 to 8.3 percent in 1975.

However, the great expectations held out for hospital rate setting are not necessarily matched by programmatic capabilities for meeting them. It would be a highly complex and delicate task to set payment rates at the point where the nation's approximately 7,000 diverse hospitals would be neither overpaid, to the detriment of the public purse, nor underpaid, to the detriment of the public well-being. Although nine state governments have established some form of hospital rate setting or rate review procedure since 1969, and 22 Blue Cross plans now reimburse their member hospitals on the basis of prospectively determined rates or charges, the state of the art is still rudimentary. At best, results so far have been equivocal.

Impeded Progress

Progress in refining rate setting processes has been seriously impeded by the lack of good data on which to base rate setting decisions, to review hospital appeals for adjustments, and to evaluate program accomplishments. Although good information will never be able to guarantee a good rate setting process, poor information does guarantee a poor one. Access to appropriate information of good quality is essential if hospital rates are to be set equitably in a manner that is administratively feasible and that promotes the achievement of overall health system objectives. In its absence, at least two types of unfortunate consequences are predictable:

1. The rate setting process will either be inequitable or will be inordinately complex, slow, and expensive, opening the administering agency to justifiable criticism from providers and the public, expressed in appeals, litigation, and political actions.
2. The potential of rate setting to improve the cost-effectiveness of health care delivery will be lost. Worse, in efforts to simplify the process, rate setters may come to rely on some grossly inadequate data just because it is easily available.

Identifying Needs

In Section 1533(d) of the 1974 Planning Act, requiring the development of uniform accounting and reporting, Congress has sought to remedy one basic weakness in the information presently available for rate setting. Various state commissions and Blue Cross plans are also beginning to find ways around some other perhaps equally important barriers to securing and using necessary information of requisite quality. However, for the most part, the data base for rate setting is not adequate for the uses to which it must be put.

In anticipation of the federal government's likely future involvement in this new form of regulatory activity, in February 1975 the Office of Research and Statistics of the Social Security Administration contracted with the Harvard Center for Community Health and Medical Care to identify the major types of information problems encountered by some of the ongoing rate setting programs and to report what is being done or what might be done to alleviate them. The purpose was to explicate some of the issues involved in improving the information base for rate setting and program monitoring and to make recommendations that might be useful to SSA or other agencies involved in writing regulations or specifying guidelines for possible future federal rate setting legislation. The observations in this article draw, in large part, from the findings of this study. Those who wish more detail are referred to working papers from this project, listed in the Appendix.

The first and soundest principle governing the collection of data is that they be tailored exactly to the purposes for which they are to be used. The tremendous masses of duplicative, uncoordinated, untimely, and often unused data that hospitals supply to various regulatory bodies and third party payers attest to the fact that this principle is honored far more in the breach than in the observance. Hospital rate setting programs, however, probably have a better excuse than do most other types of agencies since they represent a new form of regulatory activity. Few were in operation before 1971. Thus, their goals, their processes of administration, and their corresponding requirements for data are still changing markedly from year to year. Furthermore, unless premature federal legislation and regulations should impose a straitjacket on their future evolution, an even faster pace of change seems likely over the next five or ten years.

Writing in 1976, it would be foolhardy to try to specify the particular elements of any one data set to meet rate setters' needs in the years to come. Instead, this article reviews the kinds of information that state and Blue Cross rate setting programs currently employ, notes some changing perceptions of the kind of information that they may seek in the future, and then summarizes the broad types of information that would appear to be desirable to have should Congress enact hospital rate setting legislation either for the Medicare program and/or for national health insurance. Questions of the quality of the data and obstacles to their availability are discussed only in passing.

INFORMATION USED BY CURRENT RATE SETTING PROGRAMS

Major Types of Data

Three global types of consideration shape the choices on information presently used in the prospective establishment of hospital rates: first, the requirements of the particular reimbursement method being employed; second, the cost containment goals, both stated and unstated, of the agency administering the program; and third, the availability of the data desired.

Reimbursement aspects will not be considered at length here—the types of information necessary to permit distinguishing between allowable and unallowable costs under different third parties' principles of payment, the allocation of costs through cost finding, cost proportionment among different payers, reports and approvals to comply with Section 1122, and similar requirements. These issues have been covered by other publications in this series.[1] However, the fact that reimbursement methods in current use by most third parties already require extensive reports of costs and volumes of activity and of the financial feasibility of new projects means that rate setters usually start off with the potential for securing a large core of financial and statistical data that hospitals have long been accustomed to report. The detailed categorization of these data depends on the type of payment unit employed—per diem or charges—and planning agency requirements. By the same token, however, the exigencies of the reimbursement method strongly influence the scope and character of the financial data that are easily accessible to rate setters.

Changes in the reporting of costs and the additions of the many other types of data that rate setters wish to employ are dictated by their particular program goals and the particular methodologies that they choose to employ. This section outlines information needs from that perspective, drawing on the project's studies of information used by various states and Blue Cross plans.

In summary, we will discover that programs presently use or have immediate plans to use the following major types of data for budget reviews and rate setting:

1. Financial statements, fund balances, costs and revenues (historical and projected), matched to volumes of services, activities, and manpower and supply inputs.
2. Scope of services—bed capacity by service, special services, ancillary and other; physician characteristics; education programs.
3. Burden of illness brought to hospital—diagnostic case mix, case complexity, patient characteristics, procedures performed.
4. Planning data—hospital service area population characteristics, resources available to populations in specific geographic areas, and hospitalization rates.
5. Economic indicators.

Some programs use almost all these types of data; others use only a limited proportion. New programs employ the widest range. A few programs also try to factor into their rate setting decisions information concerning appropriateness of utilization (lengths of stays, underutilized high technology services) and quality of care (accreditation only).

Information Needs Geared to Program Objectives

The types of information and level of detail that rate setters require depend on the objectives of their particular program. Though the recent push toward hospital rate setting has been primarily fueled by the public's and third party payers' concern with containing hospital cost increases, different rate setting programs currently interpret their cost control mission in quite different ways. For some, rate setting is viewed primarily as a process for stimulating better hospital management that, in turn, should result in lower costs; for the majority the task is to control hospital prices for given units of services, e.g., per diem rates or charges. A few programs, perhaps in the vanguard, seek to impose annual limits on total hospital revenues both within hospitals and within a geographic region and, thus, to force better resource allocation practices both within and among its institutions. In addition, laws and contracts can give the program other responsibilities, such as meeting a hospital's full financial requirements and fair share payment to all payers. From interviews with officials of state programs and various Blue Cross plans it is apparent that most try to steer a safe course that will satisfy all such objectives to a greater or lesser degree, in the light of local perceptions of where potential hospital cost excesses lie and the points

Though the recent push toward hospital rate setting has been primarily fueled by the public's and third party payers' concern with containing hospital cost increases, different rate setting programs currently interpret their cost control mission in quite different ways.

at which it is technically and politically feasible to try to control them.

These perceptions may, and do, change over time in response to fiscal pressures on the state or Blue Cross plan and actions by consumers and hospital groups. Until now, the thrust has been to improve hospital efficiency, acting on the implied assumption that important excess costs stem from fat in hospital budgets, underutilization of facilities, and/or poor management. To identify this presumptive fat, the principal emphasis has been on analysis of labor and supply costs, using discovery of outlier situations to scale down hospital first-round demands for price increases.

Almost all rate setting programs also try to use the rate structure to curb unnecessary expansion of hospital facilities and duplication of programs. Apart from these few general characteristics, the nation's rate setting or rate review programs are highly diverse. To bring some sort of order to this diversity, William Dowling has introduced the useful concept of different generations of rate setting programs.[2] Although they have evolved in more or less historical sequence, programs typifying each generation are now operating concurrently in various parts of the nation. Each has its own type of data needs. Some programs incorporate features of several generations.

THE RATE SETTING GENERATIONS

The first generation programs, of which the Indiana Blue Cross program is the prototype, concentrate on budget reviews of individual hospitals. They are designed to spot excessive year-to-year changes in the operating costs of hospital departments and to spot management inefficiencies, particularly in the hotel-type support services of hospitals.[3] They rely on peer disclosure and persuasion to influence the behavior of administrators and trustees. Most of the programs are conducted under terms of Blue Cross contracts and are, therefore, to a greater or lesser extent voluntary, i.e., hospitals can withdraw from Blue Cross participation if they are dissatisfied with the results. In some cases, hospital trustee representatives and administrators serve on the budget review committees; trustees might also be asked to attend reviews of their own hospital's budget. Hospitals submit financial statements to the reviewers together with a package of standard forms and schedules designed for the purpose. The information about hospital costs and volumes of activity that the programs require is usually similar to that required on the Medicare cost report, the 40-page package of schedules and worksheets completed annually by all hospitals participating in the Medicare program; but they may request more or less detail.

Some programs ask for reports based on the hospitals' prior year actual costs and volumes of activity, some for current year estimates. These historical cost data from the hospitals are juxtaposed to budgets that project costs and volumes for the coming year according to the same categories, enabling the reviewers to monitor changes.

With one exception that will be noted, this same basic model of cost and budget report submissions underlies all the other rate setting generation programs. However, the first generation programs are unique in not attempting to use their reports for comparative analysis. Recognizing the difficulties of obtaining comparable data occasioned by hospital accounting organized solely to serve the purposes of internal management, they confine their analysis to the cost trend experience in each individual hospital.

Second generation rate setting, exemplified by the state and Blue Cross programs in New York state, focuses almost solely on keeping hospitals' per diem rate increases in line with the rate of overall economic inflation. In addition to promote efficiency, hospitals are penalized if the occupancy rates of various services fall below certain prescribed minimums. Unlike any of the other rate setting generations, no hospital budgets are submitted; prices are calculated under formulas that rely entirely on historical cost data (a base year of audited actual costs and a current year of nine months actual and three months estimated). The Uniform Cost Report the hospitals submit is similar to that of the first generation programs, but a companion Uniform Statistical Report yields considerably more detail on size, location, type of control, and teaching status variables. These are used to construct comparison hospital groups. The programs also employ a variety of economic data, largely derived from government reports, to construct economic change indexes.

Third generation programs, such as in Maryland and New Jersey, lay prime stress on improving hospital productivity and rely heavily on comparative analysis of both costs and budgets, using computer screens. They base a considerable portion of their comparative analysis on direct costs per unit of service, both according to hospital departments and to prescribed, defined cost centers before allocation of indirect costs. Since such analyses cannot be performed reliably in the absence of uniform accounting and reporting, this type of program usually mandates the adoption of such new systems. They require a far greater wealth of detail than is sought by the first and second generation programs. See Table 7-1 for a list of schedules in the Maryland program. It is an evolving process that Dowling describes as follows:[2]

> Once the reviewers have obtained the basic cost data, they decide that they need more detail and begin to ask the hospitals to relate their inputs to departments, to permit comparison between hospitals. The next stage is to recognize that total costs are not enough. They then begin to look at cost per unit of service in different cost centers. This requires still more data. Then the rate setter realizes that since costs are primarily a function of one particular type of input—manhours—he needs better breakdowns of manhours by department or cost center. Then, since costs are manhours times the compensation for these manhours, he begins to seek detailed data on salary levels and fringe benefits to relate to the unit costs.

In addition, the programs usually add schedules to their cost and budget report packages that will reveal details on particular areas of suspected high costs,

TABLE 7-1
Forms Required in Hospital Submissions to the Maryland Health Services Cost Review Commission

Schedule	Title
UBS	Balance Sheet—Unrestricted Funds
RBS	Balance Sheet—Restricted Funds
SFB	Statement of Changes in Equity
RE	Statement of Income and Expense
FP	Statement of Changes in Financial Position
A	Gross Operating Revenues
B	Fringe Benefits
I-1	FTEs—General Service, Auxiliary Enterprises, and Other Institutional Programs
I-2	FTEs—Patient Care Centers
MS	Room and Daily Patients Care Center Statistics
NS	Ancillary and Outpatient Care Center Statistics
R	Hospital-Based Physicians
DR	Dealings and Relationships with Certain Entities
OO	Data Concerning Owners and Related Organizations
	Budget Schedules
V-1	Forecasts of the Number of Inpatients and the Number of Patient Days
V-2	Forecasts of the Number of Outpatient Visits
V-3	Bases for Budgeting Ancillary Service Units
V-4	Computation of Volume Changes
V-5	EQUIVALENT INPATIENT DAYS*
W	New Programs
S	Summary of Internal Budget Adjustments
C	GENERAL SERVICE CENTER BUDGETS
CWS	Service Center Worksheet
CC-1	Cafeteria
CC-2	Cafeterial Loss Treated as Fringe Benefit
CU	Energy Cost Center
D	PATIENT SERVICE CENTERS
E	AUXILIARY ENTERPRISES (AE)
F	OTHER INSTITUTIONAL PROGRAMS (OIP)
J	General Service Cost Apportionment
H-1	Building Facility Allowance
H-2	Departmental Movable Equipment Allowance
H-3	Distribution of Capital Facilities Allowance
H-4	CAPITAL FACILITY ALLOWANCE SUMMARY
H-5	Buildings/Equipment Fund Statement of Changes in Fund Balances
G	Other Financial Considerations
GR	Cash and Marketable Assets
GT	Charity and Bad Debt Allowances
K	Summary of Auxiliary Enterprises
L	Summary of Other Institutional Programs
M	PATIENT SERVICE CENTER SUMMARY
PD-1	Third Party Payer Differential
MA	RATE SUMMARY AND COMPARISONS

*Major Schedules are in capital letters

such as compensation of radiologists, pathologists and consultants, leasing arrangements, and, for profit-making hospitals, payments to owners and relatives.

A fourth generation, exemplified by the Blue Cross of Western Pennsylvania and the Washington state programs, also relies heavily on comparative analysis of direct costs by cost centers, but it takes into account a wide variety of other factors in addition to management efficiency that can influence these differences. They exercise great care in constructing their hospital groups for comparative analysis, explicitly seeking to factor in differences in the hospitals' scope of services, the degree of specialization of their medical staffs, the extent and character of their education programs, and the nature of the populations they serve. This calls for each hospital to report its physician roster, its medical programs, and its teaching programs in considerable detail, either on separate schedules of the cost or budget report, or through special surveys. Table 7-2 shows the level of detail the Washington program requires of physician staff.

Finally, the most advanced generation programs are apt to be concerned with total expenditures for hospital care in their area, rather than simply with unit prices. This can take the form of limits on volume increases as well as prices, as in recent efforts of the Connecticut commission, or of some stated ceiling limit on total hospital expenditures for a geographic area, as in the Rhode Island Blue Cross plan's MAXICAP, within which individual hospitals' budgets are negotiated.

Program Trends

Regardless of generation, most rate setting programs closely monitor trends in the financial status of the hospitals in their jurisdiction or plan area, their cash flow position, and net margins. Many actively seek to minimize hospitals' dependence on short term loans. To a greater or lesser degree the programs also try to anticipate hospitals' future capital requirements by asking for three- to five-year capital budgets. Some programs also ask hospitals to furnish narrative statements describing their present and future missions and short and long term objectives.

Most rate setting programs actively seek to prevent or reduce excess bed capacity and duplication of services. This has led to increasingly strong working relationships between rate setters and certificate of need agencies in reviewing the appropriateness of proposed new capital spending and/or new medical programs. At a minimum, most programs now seek data by which to determine the impact of such proposed expansions on future operating costs, as well as on the capital costs of hospitals, and require information that justifies the support of such new costs in the future rate structure. This might call for detailed analysis of architectural plans and construction estimates and costs. A variety of other special studies might be required to determine anticipated changes in operating costs and revenues, especially for high technology services such as CAT scanners. Finally, the responses to appeals and litigations that

TABLE 7-2
The Washington State Hospital Commission's Schedule on Physician Staff

Budget Period From ________ To ________

Hospital ________________ Address ________________

License No. ________ Administrator ________________ Phone ( ) ________ Date Submitted ________

1a.

Line No.	Clinical Specialty	*Active Medical Staff Profile MD's/DO's (Enter No.): Hospital Based: Board Certified A	Hospital Based: Board Eligible B	Hospital Based: Other C	Non-Hospital Based: Board Certified D	Non-Hospital Based: Board Eligible E	Non-Hospital Based: Other F	Intern/Resident Profile (Enter No.): Approved Programs: Intern G	Approved Programs: Extern H	Approved Programs: Resident I	Other Residents J
01	Family Practice										
02	General Practice										
03	OB/GYN										
04	Pediatrics										
05	Psychiatry										
06	Oncology										
07	General Surgery										
08	Neurosurgery										
09	Thoracic Surgery										
10	Urology										
11	Cardiovascular Surgery										
12	Plastic Surgery										
13	Orthopedic Surgery										
14	Vascular Surgery										
15	Oral Surgery										
16	Internal Medicine										
17	Cardiology										
18	Gastroenterology										
19	Neurology										
20	Ophthalmology										
21	Dermatology										
22	Endocrinology										
23	Hematology										
24	Anesthesiology										
25	Radiology										
26	Pathology										
27	Podiatry										
28	Dental										
29	TOTAL										

*Beginning of Budget Year.

hospitals bring requires the ad hoc collection of data relevant to the issue at hand.

One should also note the possible sources of excess hospital costs that rate setters have so far studiously *avoided* attempting to control. High on the list stands inappropriate patient management: unnecessary admissions, unnecessary surgery and/or other services and procedures, and iatrogenic complications. Even when utilization review systems and medical audits are functioning in an area, no systematic communication between the two types of external reviewers has been established. Although they well recognize that physicians are responsible for the largest share of cost-generating decisions in hospitals, rate setters are loath to take actions that might be interpreted as interfering with physician prerogatives. Only one program, that of Rhode Island Blue Cross, seeks to moderate excessive lengths of patient stay.

One should also note the possible sources of excess hospital costs that rate setters have so far studiously* avoided *attempting to control: unnecessary admissions, unnecessary surgery and/or other services and procedures, and iatrogenic complications.

Program Objectives

In summary, to advance toward whichever broad cost containment goals they choose to pursue, most rate setting bodies have adopted one or more of the following types of programmatic objectives, using their rate setting powers at some point in the process.

Establish macroeconomic controls:

- limits on overall price or revenue increases for individual hospitals;
- limits on overall expenditure increases for hospitals within a defined geographic area.

Encourage better management:

- via the budget review process itself;
- via microcontrols on allowable unit cost increases in specific hospital departments or cost centers.

Discourage underutilization:

- direct penalties on low occupancy services;
- indirect penalties via microcontrols on unit costs.

Rationalize facility and program expansions:

- provide cost analyses for certificate of need reviews and require planning and CON approvals before considering rate adjustments;
- independently calculate costs and benefits in determining rate adjustments for expansions.

Encourage better patient management:

- discourage excessive lengths of stay (Rhode Island only).

Table 7-3 sets forth some of the types of cost and other data that eight different states and Blue Cross rate setting programs employ to pursue these objectives. The listings are not intended to be in any way inclusive; nor do all the example programs use the same types of data in pursuing the same objective. However, the table does illustrate the range and

TABLE 7-3

Rate Setting Objectives Related to Types of Data Employed in Eight Selected State and Blue Cross Programs, 1976*

Large Objective	Intermediate Objectives	Rate Setting Program Examples*	Types of Data That Can Be Used
Macrocontrol	Keep hospital cost increases in line with inflation increases.	New York, Massachusetts (for Medicaid), Western Pennsylvania Blue Cross — formula application; Arizona, Maryland, New Jersey, Rhode Island Blue Cross — nonformula	• Historic costs, rate projections, related to economic indexes constructed from data from: —Consumer Price Index —Wholesale Price Index —BLS (or local) salary surveys —Actual price trends in certain items, e.g., fuel, malpractice insurance, etc. —Proxies for other supply items —Wage and salary trend proxies, etc.
	Keep hospital cost increases in line with peer group averages	Western Pennsylvania Washington New York	• Grouping schemes might use data including the following: —Number of licensed beds; patient days —Urban/nonurban locations —Approved teaching programs; interns, residents —Number, mix of board certified specialists —Number and type of special services, weighted by imputed costs —Age, income characteristics of population in hospital service area —Proportion of Medicare days to total days
	Keep hospitals solvent but restrict revenue margin.	Arizona Washington Massachusetts Rhode Island Indiana Blue Cross Maryland New Jersey	• Financial statements • Fund balance changes • Net margins • Cash budgets, collectables; contractual allowances, bad debts
	Individual hospital rate increases calculated within a set maximum expenditure increase for the geographic region.	Rhode Island New Jersey (capital expenditures)	• Bottom line projected increases all hospitals in geographic region • Capital spending needs for region

*The programs used as illustrations in this exhibit are: Arizona, Indiana Blue Cross, Maryland, Massachusetts, New Jersey, New York, Rhode Island Blue Cross, Washington, and Western Pennsylvania Blue Cross. In Rhode Island the program is cooperative between Blue Cross and the state; in New York the state administers rate setting for Medicaid and establishes the regulatory framework within which eight Blue Cross plans administer rate setting formulas and submit rate recommendations for approval by state agencies. Arizona's program is solely for mandatory rate review; the state has no authority to establish rates.

TABLE 7-3
(*Continued*)

Large Objective	Intermediate Objectives	Rate Setting Program Examples*	Types of Data That Can Be Used
Encourage Better Management	Encourage better internal accountability of hospital departments	New Jersey (before 1974) Washington Rhode Island (Blue Cross) Western Pennsylvania Blue Cross Indiana (Blue Cross) Most other Blue Cross rate-setting programs	• Cost and budget reports, reporting and review process designed to: encourage better budgeting procedures, internal reporting systems; display aberrant departmental cost increases, staffing patterns, etc., to hospital administrators, trustees; encourage physicians to prioritize new spending demands, e.g., emphasize use of data for internal hospital purposes.
	Encourage management by objectives	Washington Maryland	• Statement by each department of particular cost savings objectives for budget year and imputed dollar savings; statement of total hospital cost-saving objectives, imputed dollar savings. Checks with actual achievement following year.
	Identify inefficiencies in hospital operations by statistical analysis, exception reviews of unit costs and display, penalize internal cross subsidies.	Arizona Maryland Washington New Jersey (1976) Rhode Island	• Detailed reports of costs, revenues, volumes by cost centers. (Requires uniform accounting and reporting, reclassification of responsibility cost centers to functional activity centers for comparative analysis of direct unit costs matched to revenues before and after allocation of indirect costs.)
	Discover and disclose the compensation rates of hospital-based physicians.	Arizona Maryland New York (selective) New Jersey Western Pennsylvania Washington	• Reports on physician compensation arrangements, duties, and hours.
	Detect conflict of interest situations	New York Maryland Washington New Jersey Arizona	• Statements on hospital transactions with business in which board members or officers have financial interest.

TABLE 7-3
(Continued)

Large Objective	Intermediate Objectives	Rate Setting Program Examples*	Types of Data That Can Be Used
Discourage Under-Utilization	Penalize underutilized services to encourage phaseouts, e.g., obstetrics, pediatrics, etc.	New York Massachusetts Rhode Island New Jersey	• Beds, admissions, patient days by type of hospital service—calculation of occupancy rates
	Penalize underutilized high technological procedures, e.g., open heart surgery, dialysis, etc., to encourage phaseouts	New York	• Number of procedures per year of specified types related to number of deaths by patient age.
Rationalize Hospital Expansions	Discourage new medical programs, new facilities, new major equipment or replacements not needed by the population in the hospital's service area. (Need determination from planning or CON bodies).	Arizona Massachusetts New York Maryland New Jersey Rhode Island Washington Western Pennsylvania Indiana	• CON agency recommendations (all programs) • Hospital service area delineation • Planning agency recommendations according to a preagreed priority ranking of needs • Long term capital budgets from hospitals • Hospital statement of mission, planning priorities (overall, and by department) • Population and resource data from planning agency staff, and staff cooperation in community need/cost impact analyses • Travel time estimates
	Encourage needed new programs, especially for alternatives to inpatient care	Washington Rhode Island New Jersey	• Planning agency priority rankings in relation to resources of hospital service area, population characteristics
Encourage Better Patient Management	Penalize excessive lengths of stay for selected diagnostic categories, age-adjusted	Rhode Island	• Hospital discharge abstract summaries (PAS)
Factor Quality Differences into Rate Decisions	Exclude hospitals with low costs associated with substandard quality from group averages	New York	• Reports from certification agencies • JCAH accreditation status

types of data that current rate setting programs find necessary to secure for accomplishing their purposes.

RELATION OF DATA AVAILABILITY TO METHODOLOGY

Common Methodologies

The types of data that are needed for implementing these widely disparate types of goals must also meet the requirements of the particular methodologies their rate setting programs employ to move toward them. The most common methodologies for reaching decisions on allowed prospective hospital operating rates are:

1. individual hospital cost and budget reviews,
2. exception reviews of peer group hospitals,
3. formula applications either for individual hospitals or for hospital groups to project allowable rates of increase in line with economic indices, and
4. special review of rates necessary to support new capital and operating costs associated with changes in facility and medical programs.

Conversely, the rate setting methodology often is shaped to accommodate the type and character of data that happen to be available when the program goes into effect. Few of the basic reporting systems that hospital rate setting bodies employ were especially designed to serve purposes of rate setting geared to cost containment and/or improvement in hospital cost effectiveness. Rather, most of them are simply outgrowths of the Medicare Cost Report and similar cost reports developed by the individual Blue Cross plans to serve as the basis for cost-based reimbursement. Some early programs of prospective reimbursement were viewed as merely shifting the time frame of payment decisions, on the assumption that this would in itself modify hospital cost increases.[3] Therefore, the original cost report models were initially seen to be basically satisfactory.

Equally important, hospitals had long become accustomed to assembling the considerable data required for their third party cost reports, and in any event they will have to continue doing so for Medicare and any other major payers not covered by the new rate setting plan. Thus to avoid duplication of hospital effort, even the newest programs' cost and budget report packages are intentionally designed in close conformity with traditional cost report categories. In Massachusetts and the New York Blue Cross plans, as in many other Blue Cross plans, the same hospital cost report serves the dual functions of reimbursement and rate setting.

No Time for New Design

Although, in theory, state rate setting programs can require hospitals to furnish any data they need, rate setting programs are usually conceived by legislators in a hurry to get action. The new administering agency is given scant time to design and set in place the type of information infrastructure it might have wanted. For example, in 1969 the New

York state legislature allowed only four months between enactment of the new rate setting law and its required implementation. There was no choice but to build the new program around the hospital cost reporting system already in place. Here, although hospitals had long used standard reporting forms, because of their widely differing internal organizational structures, they defined departmental categories and many important data elements—such as "FTEs" and "clinic visits" in a highly unstandardized fashion—preventing valid interinstitutional comparisons. A few states, however, have had the luxury of approaching rate setting in a more deliberate fashion, allowing the *de nova* design of good supporting data systems. In California, for example, a new uniform chart of accounts, then a uniform reporting system, and finally a uniform budget report system were designed, tested, and implemented; and a means for securing statewide hospital patient data from uniform hospital discharge abstracts was developed—all before rate setting legislation was enacted. (A rate setting bill is currently before the legislature.)

The Washington and Arizona programs have been able to capitalize on the developmental work in California. With a few modifications to suit local needs, they have adopted the new chart of accounts and the uniform reporting and budgeting systems almost wholesale. This greatly improves their capability for obtaining comparable data according to functional cost centers.

The almost universal lack of 100 percent reporting of hospital patient data from uniform hospital discharge systems has profoundly influenced the character of hospital rate setting programs to date. Patient case mix differences have been shown to be highly correlated with differences in hospital costs.[4,5] For example, a study of cost functions in the hospitals of two Canadian provinces, Ontario and British Columbia, showed that case mix and patient age variables together explained more than 80 percent of their cost differences.[6] However, without access to relevant data, U.S. rate reviewers have been unable to take these factors into systematic account. This is one reason for the current heavy emphasis on analysis of costs related to differences in hospital inputs rather than product.

The almost universal lack of 100 percent reporting of hospital patient data from uniform hospital discharge systems has profoundly influenced the character of hospital rate setting programs to date.

Level of Detail Required

With each successive generation of rate setting programs the cost and budget packages the hospitals submit to the rate reviewers swells. The budget package submitted to the newest state rate setting program, the Washington State Hospital Commission, for example, includes 182 pages of forms on a total of 44 schedules. However, lest this reporting burden on hospitals be considered self-evidently outrageous, one should note that appeals and lawsuits brought by Washington hospitals are almost nonexistent, compared with those from hospitals in New York. In this, the oldest state program, hospitals are required to fill out a mere 56 pages on the two required reports, the Uniform Financial Report (UFR) and the Uniform Statistical Report (USR). In hospital rate setting, at least with today's methodologies, the currently popular KISS acronym—Keep It Simple Stupid—seems less relevant than the more venerable adage which reminds us that simplicity is the enemy of equity. Most hospitals, if their costs are to be compared with those of other hospitals, prefer to supply increasingly detailed data rather than to risk arbitrary decisions resulting from a reviewer's calculations based on highly aggregated data.

"Hospitals are being averaged to death," one hospital spokesman recently observed. Until recently, for example, New York's Uniform Financial Report divided natural expenses into only two categories: salary and nonsalary. Frustrated in attempts to find explanations of wide differences in the operating costs of their departments as reported on the UFR, in 1975 a committee of hospital financial officers and Blue Cross officials proposed a drastic expansion that would have reported 49 categories of nonlabor expense and 10 categories of labor expense.

Although rate setting programs might recognize that fine-grained data are required to make complex decisions on hospital rates and although hospitals might be compliant in supplying such data, practical constraints of budget and staff pose limits on the amount that can be actually edited, verified, processed, analyzed, and interpreted. The development of even more sophisticated classification schemes and economic indices could, in the future, offer partial solutions to this problem. However, devising methodologies that will yield classification schemes and indices that are fair to both payers and providers is a difficult task. No one claims to have found satisfactory solutions. Still, serious developmental work is underway in several programs.

"Hospitals are being averaged to death," one hospital spokesman recently observed.

Data for Hospital Grouping

Given the extraordinary diversity in the hospital industry, ranging from cottage hospitals to enormous multifunction medical centers, a wide range of characteristics must be accounted for if the hospitals are to be classified into homogeneous comparison groups. Such variables must be chosen to reflect properly the important characteristics both of the hospitals themselves and of the particular social and economic environment in which they operate. As an illustration, the variables used to construct comparison groups through cluster analysis for the 119 hospitals in the state of Washington include:

1. available beds,
2. licensed beds,
3. nonprofit/profit,
4. nongovernment/government,
5. accreditation status,
6. service index (constructed to take account of the proportion of spe-

cial services the hospital offers weighted according to relative cost),
7. interns,
8. residents,
9. physician mix index (constructed to take account of the proportion of board certified specialists on the hospitals' staffs, based on data supplied in Table 7-2),
10. hospital beds per 1000 population in the hospital survey area,
11. physicians per 1000 population in area,
12. median income of the population in area,
13. percent urban population in area, and
14. percent of population 65 years or over in area.

There are several other advanced classification schemes, notably the point predictive method employed in prospective rate setting by the Blue Cross of Western Pennsylvania, and the American Hospital Association's classification, from which the Washington system was modeled, that employs 21 variables.[7,8] In contrast cruder classifications, such as that employed by SSA for Medicare cost, limits accounts for only three or four factors, such as bed size, urban/rural location, and some gross measure of the economic status of a large geographic area. Such systems are notable for the volume of appeals and litigations they inspire.

Data for Economic Indices

Similarly, a wide range of detailed economic data are required to construct indices to project some allowable percentage increase in hospital rates that will equitably account for increases in expenses due to changes in the prices of goods and services required to produce hospital care. Since national or statewide economic indicators in no way reflect local conditions, the sensitivity of the economic index depends in large part on both the availability of sound proxies for the prices of goods and services in subareas of a state or region and the willingness and ability of the rate setting program to use them. Rate setting programs differ considerably in these respects. The New Jersey program, for example, employs only two proxies and two weights to represent all hospital goods and services, i.e., the Bureau of Labor Statistics Consumer Price Index is taken as proxy for changes in the prices of almost all nonsalary items (a few, such as malpractice insurance, are considered totally out of the hospital's control and are specifically designated as passthroughs); the Bureau of Labor Statistics Average Hourly Earnings of Manufacturing Employees in New Jersey is taken as proxy for wage and salary changes of all hospital employees. This index is currently under challenge by New Jersey hospitals as being too gross to yield accurate predictions of trends in hospital input prices.[9]

ELABORATE INDICES

The New York State programs, on the other hand, have elaborate indices that are continually being tested and refined.[10] For example, the index used in New York City in 1975 employed 44 proxies for 10 categories of wage and salary items and 20 proxies for 40 categories of nonlabor items. Between these extremes, the index used for setting Medicaid rates in Massachusetts employs 14 indices for nonsalary items and 4 categories for salaries and wages. The latter distinguishes between movements in compensation of top professionals and administrators, middle management, technical and skilled, and unskilled workers.

INDIVIDUALLY APPLIED INDICES

The Massachusetts index appears to be well received by both the Rate Setting Commission and the hospitals, possibly because it is applied individually to each hospital. Recognizing that the labor component can run from 60 to 75 percent of the total operating costs of any given institution, it weights the distribution of labor and nonlabor costs according to the hospital's actual historical experience. Had the same index been applied statewide to all hospitals or to hospitals in grossly classified groups, it might have been heavily criticized. This illustrates, once again, that the level of detail required depends on the application of all methodological components of any particular rate setting system.[11]

CHANGING PERSPECTIVES OF DATA NEEDS

Although the previous section has suggested the major types of data used to meet the needs perceived by state and Blue Cross hospital rate setters in 1976, it probably does not project what their data needs will be in 1980. In hospital rate setting, change is the name of the game. Almost every program studied was rethinking or expanding its objectives, experimenting with new rate setting methods, or refining older ones. Equally important, programs are also rethinking their relationships with certificate of need bodies and future HSAs, in response to the terms of P.L. 93-641 and PSRO legislation. Some of these changes reflect the realization that, in the absence of meaningful measures of differences in the nature of the services that hospitals actually produce, current attempts to measure "productivity" in hospitals are at best quixotic; at worst, dangerous. New ways are being sought to analyze cost differences in relation both to differences in the complexity of these services and to differences in patient mix. Other changes could be coming in response to challenges to improve the cost effectiveness of hospital services in relation to the population's health needs—raising fundamental questions as to differences in utilization and patient management practices, and the role of reinbursement in helping secure the best value for the health dollars society spends.

In the absence of meaningful measures of differences in the nature of the services that hospitals actually produce, current attempts to measure "productivity" in hospitals are at best quixotic; at worst, dangerous.

Differences in the Nature of Hospital Activities

Rate setters have been frustrated in trying to develop objective standards of hospital efficiency that they can use to make impartial rate decisions which will not overpay some hospitals for the type and quality of the work they do while underpaying others. Hospitals that stand to lose from rate decisions based on comparative screens are quick to point out in detail why their costs are higher than average. Standards of performance efficiency must be able to withstand the test of appeals and legal challenges, yet the statistical bases on which hospital performance is measured are widely recognized to be inadequate.

TRADITIONAL CHART OF ACCOUNTS

With a few exceptions, the traditional measures set forth in the AHA Chart of Accounts in 1954 have continued to be carried forward into the two full-scale revisions of the Chart in 1964 and 1976. Simple counts of laboratory tests, for example, conceal differences in test complexity that call for widely varying mixes of time, materials, and levels of technical training. Lacking any weighting to reflect such factors, a bone marrow analysis counts equally with a pap smear. The same principle pertains in many other areas of hospital performance: when operating room costs among hospitals are compared on the basis of numbers of operations performed (or operating room minutes) without weightings, an appendectomy will equal an open heart procedure—yet the support staff and equipment required are obviously of an entirely different order of magnitude. Such averaging penalizes hospitals that give complicated services requiring complicated mixes of resources, while it overpays simpler service hospitals. Rate setting bodies are becoming increasingly aware of these problems; and, encouraged by hospital associations, many are experimenting with new types of activity measures.

RELATIVE VALUE SCALES

The principle of relative value scales is looked to as one means of accounting for differences in the complexity of what hospitals do in many realms of their activities. Herkimer, for example, urges that hospitals accumulate and project all their production statistics based on relative unit values for each department, and that the denominator for judging efficiency be changed from dollars to productive manhours required.[12,13] Will Bishop has proposed a similar approach through the development of Patient Service Units (PSUs), first for all hospital ancillary departments and then for nursing care. He suggests that if a standardized reporting system for PSUs were developed and universally adopted by hospitals, the units could eventually replace the patient day as the basic measure of output, yielding a more equitable basis for comparison among hospitals as well as a better tool by which hospital management could judge the staffing efficiency of its departments.[14]

Unfortunately, only a few relative value scales have as yet been adopted. The most commonly used ones are those developed by the American College of Radiology for reporting radiological procedures and by the College of American Pathologists for reporting laboratory procedures. Most of the newer rate setting programs have incor-

TABLE 7-4
Relative Value Scales Used by Maryland's Health Services Cost Review Commission

Service Center	Type of Relative Value Unit
Laboratory	The College of American Pathologists workload recording method for clinical laboratories
Radiology, including Nuclear Medicine, Radioisotopes, Diagnostic, Therapeutic	American College of Radiologists relative value units
Pulmonary Function	Connecticut Hospital Association relative value units
EEG and EKG	California Medical Association
Physical Therapy	California Medical Association

porated these scales (see, for example, Table 7-4).

Although existing relative values scales are an improvement over simple counts of workload units, most commentators consider that far more developmental work is required if they are properly to account for differences in the time, skills, and materials that go into producing different hospital "products."[15] If rate setting is to move toward greater equity, such developmental work must go forward.

Differences in Hospital Case Mix

The most glaring gaps in information by which to compare hospital costs in relation to their performance stems from the absence of patient data. Though it is obvious that costs of care will, or should be, higher for patients with complex medical problems and for patients in vulnerable age groups, case mix and patient profiles of hospitals are rarely matched with cost profiles for purposes of rate setting. However, this situation, too, is changing. Rate setting bodies and hospitals are becoming increasingly aware of the need to account for case mix and the corresponding need to generate reports on hospitals patients from uniform discharge abstracts or other sources. Both the Maryland and New Jersey programs have issued regulations requiring hospitals to furnish patient data, and the New York and Massachusetts programs are also involved in developmental efforts. As noted earlier, Rhode Island already employs such information. This reflects the proposition that data on hospital costs, revenues, and volumes, however well reported, can give only half the hospital performance picture.

OUTPUT APPROACH

The desirability of an output approach, where payment is made according to adequate treatment of specifically defined illnesses, has long been recognized.[16] Various models and constructs have been developed. The common problem has been how to develop patient classes that take proper account of the wide range of possible diagnoses, the different degrees of morbidity and disability that are present within any given diagnostic class, the frequency of multiple diagnoses, and characteristics of patients such as age, nutritional status, etc., that influence their requirements for care and responses to treatment. Considerable work has gone forward in the development of patient classes, both for patients with acute and long term illnesses.[17,18] One such system, developed at Yale, is about to be tried by the New Jersey rate setting body on an experimental basis. John Thompson described the rationale as follows:[19]

> We assume that the control of cost is inextricably linked with the processes of patient care in terms of resource use, and rests upon understanding the patient management process as it is applied appropriately to unique classes of patients. It is not sufficient to deal with utilization review and quality of care as a process separable from the expenditure of manpower, facilities and equipment in delivering that care, or vice versa. Research is going forward to link these three elements of cost, utilization and quality to form the basis for hospital comparisons needed for rate reviews and rate setting.
>
> The critical need is for a method by which hospitals can be characterized in terms of the services they provide to patients and the resources consumed for each delivery incident. What is required is the ability to describe the unique patient care processes delivered by each hospital and to measure the costs incurred in producing this mix of services for patient care. With this approach, a state or region will be able to implement equitable rate setting, monitor hospital performance, and at the same time produce and feed back to each hospital the information it needs to review and evaluate its own performance and quality criteria.

Whether this particular system actually proves feasible and can fulfill the hopes of its designers, it indicates one radically different approach to hospital rate setting that might be just down the road. Once it is recognized that it does no good to compare cost of services by hospital departments if the cases are different, and that one must adjust department costs by type of cases served and resource imputs employed to set equitable rates, the methodologies for doing so will be developed. To set rates according to such output measures would require:

1. hospital patient data describing diagnoses, procedures performed, and treatments given;
2. matching financial data by cost centers;
3. protocols of treatment and/or criteria, such as those recently developed under contract with HEW's Bureau of Quality Assurance, by which other reviewers could assess the quality of care.

It is interesting to note that in Quebec, where hospital costs and budgets have been subject to external review since 1962, a major shift to incorporate patient data in the process is now also being planned. The Dumbaugh report found this to be the most important impending change in that province's system:[20]

> . . .where users initially were satisfied to

judge hospital performance on unit costs/activity centers . . . now the number of services consumed by the patient in each diagnostic category is considered information necessary for control purposes. Expanding the information system so that it can accommodate such frequent demand for patient data is one of the projects of [the Ministry]. The present patient discharge summary form does provide diagnostic data, but no information on the services consumed by each patient.

A revision of the patient data (hospital discharge abstract) form to make this possible is expected by November 1976.

Closer Attention to Utilization and to Patient Outcome

Rate setting programs that place major emphasis on lowering the unit costs of hospital services, as already noted, penalize hospitals with low occupancy rates since such hospitals have a high ratio of fixed versus variable costs. In the name of efficiency, this creates incentives to hospitals to increase their volume of services. Although unit costs might indeed go down, the end result could be to increase the total volume of expenditures by those who pay the bills. Similarly, rates calculated on budget projections will yield higher total revenues than anticipated if the hospitals' actual volume of services exceeds those that had been projected. To close such escape hatches it can be anticipated that rate setting programs will attempt to monitor hospital volume more closely during the projected rate year and to adjust rates accordingly. The Rhode Island Blue Cross program has pioneered volume adjustment methodology; it receives monthly monitoring reports of both outpatient visits and inpatient admissions and patient days by service, as well as summaries of discharges and lengths of stay from the hospitals' PAS reports.[21]

APPROPRIATENESS OF UTILIZATION PRACTICES

The next logical step will be to venture into territory heretofore out of bounds to rate setters—to question the appropriateness of utilization practices. As noted earlier, Rhode Island, with its access to patient data, is already doing so. If the pressure to contain costs is sufficiently great to force a move in this direction, rate setting programs will need to establish closer communication with PSROs, who have the responsibility for decisions on the appropriateness of admissions, procedures performed, and other patient management practices. To date no programs are known to have established formal connections with PSROs, although feelers have been put out in this direction by at least four state commissions—Connecticut, Massachusetts, Washington, and New Jersey. "For," as one rate setting program executive recently observed, "what's the use of finding out if a service is being efficiently provided if the patient doesn't need it in the first place."[22]

The next logical step will be to venture into territory heretofore out of bounds to rate setters—to question the appropriateness of utilization practices.

RELEVANT ANALYSIS OF DATA

Finally, although information to describe the quality of hospital care and patient outcomes is only rarely sought by rate programs at the present time and would be generated by other agencies as health resources become more limited and as the public begins to hold reimbursement agencies accountable for assuring the best value for health dollars spent, the present separation of utilization reviews and medical audit profiles of hospitals for hospital cost profiles could well become less sacrosanct. The 1975–76 Moreland Commission's investigations of nursing home abuses in New York, for example, specifically criticized the rate setting body for making rate decisions not related to existing certification inspection reports on poor quality of care provided.[23] The recent investigation of Medicaid mills by the Sub-Committee on Long Term Care of the Senate Committee on Aging also reprimanded Medicaid officials for divorcing considerations of the quality of patient care for reimbursement.[24]

Some reports from hospitals that now go to rate setters furnish data that can be analyzed to show aberrations in case fatality rates (see Table 7-5). So far, however, such reports are not used in hospital comparisons. Although conclusions from these data would have to be drawn with extreme caution, where fatality rates were found to be high for particular types of procedures the hospital board of trustees and rate setters could jointly commission special reviews by qualified clinical specialists, or request medical care evaluation studies by PSROs.

NEW QUESTIONS AS TO THE BEST ALLOCATION OF SCARCE RESOURCES

Some other changes could be on the way, reflecting changing perceptions of the future role of hospital rate setting itself, fostered by a new realization of the need to respond to national, state, and Blue Cross fiscal imperatives. Given the ever-rising share of health care in general, and hospital care in particular, as a percentage of the gross national product, it seems likely that some sort of ceiling limits will eventually be set. As Cumming observed, "Now the issue becomes, good services for good value—or how to get the best bang for the back out of the hospital industry."[25]

This calls for rate setting, utilization review, and certificate of need agencies to operate under common policies defining the kinds of system changes sought, such as the phasing out of particular hospitals and services in certain areas of oversupply, as was recently recommended by the Mayor's Task Force in New York City. Some policies might grow out of HSA appropriateness reviews under Section 1513 (g)(1) of P.L. 93-641. In such circumstances, the HSA, guided perhaps by reports of utilization review, licensing, and quality monitoring agencies, might identify institutions or services where continued operations do not appear to be justified; the rate setting body could then gear its actions to ease the phasing out. Conversely, when institutions propose new services or where the community's need for them is identified by planning agencies, the rate setting agency can

TABLE 7-5

Utilization and Mortality by Patient Age—Medical and Surgical Services—USR 1975

Hospital Name ______________ N.Y.S. Operating Certificate No. ______

			Medical Service					Surgical Service			
			Inpatient Services			Leave Blank		Inpatient Services			Leave Blank
Age	Sex	LINE	Discharge Patient Days	Number of Discharges	Number of Deaths	Average Length of Stay	LINE	Discharge Patient Days	Number of Discharges	Number of Deaths	Average Length of Stay
			2 1 9	2 2 0	2 2 1			2 1 9	2 2 0	2 2 1	
Under age 1	M	64					80				
	F	65					81				
1 - 14	M	66					82				
	F	67					83				
15 - 24	M	68					84				
	F	69					85				
25 - 44	M	70					86				
	F	71					87				
45 - 64	M	72					88				
	F	73					89				
65 - 74	M	74					90				
	F	75					91				
75 and over	M	76					92				
	F	77					93				
TOTAL M	M	78					94				
TOTAL F	F	79					95				
TOTAL M & F		52					53				

Source: New York State Department of Health, *Uniform Statistical Report,* 1975.

provide economic analysis, perhaps suggesting negotiated tradeoffs to keep total expenditures constant for an institution.

RECOMMENDATIONS

Looking ahead to possible future rate setting responsibilities for Medicare and/or national health insurance, it could be valuable to think broadly about the major types of information that should be sought and the rationale for its use. It would be unfortunate if present practices, which are still very much in flux, should become frozen into a pattern that might constrict future development.

Should Congress mandate rate setting, it should at the same time establish rate setting objectives. It seems likely that Congress will look to rate setting as one of a set of regulatory tools by which to control increases in overall health costs, but with the goal of doing so without either diminishing patient access to needed care or the quality and effectiveness of such care.

Relating Information to Needs

If hospital rate setting is to become part of an armamentarium of regulation with which to implement broad health policies for the nation, ideally those who set hospital rates and those who monitor the results of rate setting programs should be able to relate hospital cost information to the medical needs and demographic characteristics of both the population and of the patients served; to the nature, volume and timeliness of the services provided; to the efficiency of the service delivery; to the quality of the product; and ultimately to the consequences to patients and community in terms of health, well-being, and total expenditures. This calls for relating many different data derived from disparate sources.

Obtaining Necessary Data

Much of the data necessary for sophisticated rate setting and program monitoring can best be obtained directly in annual cost and/or budget submissions from hospitals. These are, to a great extent, merely elaborations of existing reports submitted for reimbursement purposes. However, far better measures of output are required. Other types of needed information such as from hospital uniform discharge abstracts, are already being reported by many hospitals to systems such as PAS. Thus, rate setting agencies might not greatly add to the hospitals' already

If the data collection burden is not to become intolerable, rate setters, as their future information needs grow, should attempt to spin off analyses from reporting systems already in place.

heavy data collection burden. It must be remembered that if this burden is not to become intolerable, rate setters, as their future information needs grow, should attempt to spin off analyses from reporting systems already in place. Conversely, if in a given area, rate setting collects more detailed data than do other reviewing agencies, they, too, should be willing to share their data.

REFERENCES

1. See TOPICS IN HEALTH CARE FINANCING, *Medicare Reimbursement,* 1:3, Spring 1975; and *Private Third Party Reimbursement,* 2:1, Fall 1975.
2. Bauer, *Improving Information for Hospital Rate Setting,* final report of project under HEW Contract 600-75-0142 (ORS-SSA), Appendix B. Proceedings of Advisory Committee Meeting, May 5–6, 1976.
3. Feldstein, "An Analysis of Reimbursement Plans," *Reimbursement Incentives for Hospital and Medical Care: Objectives and Alternatives,* Department of Health, Education and Welfare, Washington, D.C., United States Government Printing Office, 1968.
4. Lave, Lave, and Silverman, "A Proposal for Incentive Reimbursement for Hospitals," *Medical Care,* 11:2, March–April, 1968.
5. Feldstein and Schuttinga, *Hospital Costs in Massachusetts: A Methodological Study, Discussion Paper No. 499,* Harvard Institute for Economic Research, Cambridge, 1975.
6. Evans and Walker, "Information Theory and the Analysis of Hospital Cost Structure," *Canadian Journal of Economics,* August 1972.
7. Shuman, Wolfe, and Hardwick, "Predictive Hospital Reimbursement and Evaluation Model," *Inquiry,* 9, February 1972.
8. Philip and Iyer, "Classification of Community Hospitals, *Health Services Research,* Winter 1975.
9. Rossman *et al., Analysis of the "Economic Factor" as Incorporated into the Guidelines for the 1976 Hospital Rate Program Prepared by the State of New Jersey, Department of Health,* Management and Planning Services, Hospital Association of New York State, Inc., May 1976.
10. Bauer, *Information Available for Hospital Rate Setting in New York State,* Harvard Center for Community Health and Medical Care Report Series R-45-10, Boston, April 1976.
11. Bauer, *Information Available for Hospital Rate Setting in Massachusetts,* Harvard Center for Community Health and Medical Care Report Series R-45-9, Boston, April 1976.
12. Herkimer, "The Dollar is Obsolete for Cost Comparisons," *Hospital Financial Management,* February 1970.
13. Eberhard, Herkimer, Jr., and Uhl, "The HRU Measuring Input to Find Productivity," *Hospital Financial Management,* February 1976.
14. Bishop, "Patient Service Unity—The First Step Towards Better Comparisons," *Hospital Financial Management,* March 1972.
15. Wolfe, Shuman, and Hutton, *A Critical Review of Cost Finding Methodologies,* report to the Social Security Administration under Purchase Order 0413-76-1497, May 1976.
16. Diggs, "Patient Mix: The Missing Ingredient in Understanding Hospital Costs," *Hospital Topics,* 51: 5, May 1972.
17. Cooney, *Type of Medical Care Classification System,* Hospital Research and Educational Trust, Chicago, 1974.
18. Jones, McNitt, and Densen, "Patient Assessment: Its Use in Long Term Care Facilities," *American Health Care Association Journal,* 1:3, November 1975.
19. Thompson, Mross, and Fetter, *Case Mix and Resource Use,* Center for the Study of Health Services, Yale University Institution for Social and Policy Studies, New Haven, 1975.
20. Dumbaugh, *Hospital Information Systems in the Province of Quebec,* Harvard Center for Community Health and Medical Care Report Series R-45-2, Boston, January 1976.
21. Bauer and Clark, *Budget Reviews and Prospective Rate Setting for Rhode Island Hospitals,* Harvard Center for Community Health and Medical Care, Boston, February 1974, Appendix B.
22. Bauer, *Improving Information for Hospital Rate Setting, op. cit.,* Appendix B.
23. New York State, Moreland Act Commission on Nursing Homes and Residential Facilities, *Regulating Nursing Home Care: The Paper Tigers,* Report No. 1, October 1975.
24. Bird, "Medicaid Abuse," New York *Times,* August 30, 1976, p. 1.
25. Bauer, *Improving Information for Hospital Rate Setting, op. cit.,* Appendix B.

Appendix

List of Reports and Papers from Harvard Project on Information for Hospital Rate Setting 1975-1976

CONFERENCE REPORT

Uniform Reporting for Hospital Rate Reviews: Criteria to Guide Development and Proceedings of a 1975 Conference, Katharine G. Bauer, Principal Associate, Harvard Center for Community Health.

REVIEWS OF INFORMATION SYSTEMS

Medicare

Data Rich and Information Poor: Medicare's Resources for Prospective Rate Setting (R-45-12), Diane Rowland, Associate, Harvard Center for Community Health. Each of the record systems developed by SSA to administer or monitor the Medicare programs is briefly described. Problems of information integration and sharing within SSA are discussed, particularly as they might affect the adaptation of the data base to possible future rate setting or rate setting program monitoring needs.

Quebec

Hospital Information Systems in the Province of Quebec (R-45-2), Karin Dumbaugh, Instructor in Health Services, Harvard School of Public Health. Detailed description of the various streams of data used for hospital rate setting in Quebec, the original rationale for its collection, and evolution of the system over time, together with description of the relation of the provincial to the federal reporting systems in Canada.

Reports on Five State Rate Setting Programs

Each state report covers: relation of information collected to the rate setting program's particular objectives and process; types of data available; how the reporting systems were developed; characteristics of the reporting system; validating, managing, and using the information; data sharing with other agencies; appraisal of the present information in light of criteria; future plans. Selected schedules from the program's reporting forms are included as well as lists of output measures and natural expense classifications. An appraisal of the strengths and limitations of each information system is made in accordance with the criteria developed for the project's 1975 conference on uniform reporting.

Information Available for Hospital Rate Setting in Washington State (R-45-7), Katharine G. Bauer.

Information Available for Rate Setting in Maryland (R-45-8), Katharine G. Bauer.

Information Available for Hospital Rate Setting in Massachusetts (R-45-9), Katharine G. Bauer.

Information Available for Hospital Rate Setting in New York State (R-45-10), Katharine G. Bauer.

Information Available for Hospital Rate Review in Arizona (R-45-13), Diane Rowland.

QUESTIONS OF INFORMATION INTEGRATION AND USE

The Uses of Population-Based Data for Rate Setting (R-45-5), Jennifer Robbins, Consultant to Project. The potential for linking related hospital cost and utilization data to population data to produce comparative rates for different geographic areas is explored. Such exercises are necessary to raise questions on the relation of hospitals' costs, equity of access, and appropriateness and effectiveness of care.

The Transition to Uniform Accounting and Reporting for Hospitals: Some Perspectives from Participants (R-45-13), Diane Rowland. Case examples in California and Washington illustrate the types of problems that are encountered in a statewide shift to a new hospital accounting and reporting system, and the report discusses various ways by which the transition period might be made easier.

Connections Between Rate Setting and Planning in Maryland and Rhode Island (R-45-6), Drew Altman, Department of Political Science, Massachusetts Institute of Technology. The study describes formal and informal connections between rate setting and planning agencies in Maryland and Rhode Island revealed in practices of their information use. It notes features of local history and organizational structure that appear to have influenced the notably different strengths of these connections in the two states.

Exchanges of Information Between Hospital Rate Setting and Certificate of Need Agencies: Selected State Experiences (R-45-14), Jonathan B. Brown, Diane Rowland, and Margaret Sweetland.

Disclosure of PSRO Information to Hospital Rate Setting Bodies: A Legal Analysis (R-45-1), Alan Strasser, Harvard Law School. The April 1975 PSRO draft provisions on disclosure are analyzed in respect to possible limitations on the use of PSRO data by state rate setting bodies. The disclosure questions posed are then reviewed in the context of relevant provisions of the Freedom of Information and Privacy Acts.

Living With Civil Service: The Massachusetts Experience (R-45-4), Randall Smith, Public Policy Program, Kennedy School of Government, Harvard University. Case study of civil service in Massachusetts, documenting some problems of attracting qualified professionals to state employment and suggesting ways to accommodate them.

Information Problems Experienced in Regulating Public Utilities and Parallels in Hospital Rate Setting (R-45-3), Bruce

Stangle, Sloan School, Massachusetts Institute of Technology, and Katharine G. Bauer. The literature on information problems encountered by such long established regulatory agencies as the Federal Power Commission and the Interstate Commerce Commission are reviewed, and parallels are drawn to problems encountered by hospital rate reviewers.